New Paradigms in Healthcare

In the first two decades of this new millennium, the self-sufficiency of Evidence-Based Medicine (EBM) have begun to be questioned. The narrative version gradually assumed increasing importance as the need emerged to shift to more biologically, psychologically, socially, and existentially focused models. The terrible experience of the COVID pandemic truly revealed that EBM alone, while being a wonderful scientific philosophy and containing the physician's paternalistic approach, has its limitations: it often ignores both the patient's and physician's perspectives as persons, as human beings; it pays relentless attention to biological markers and not to the more personal, psychological, social, and anthropological ones, removing the emotions, thoughts, and desires of life, focusing on just the "measurable quality" of it.

Health Humanities, Medical Humanities and Narrative Medicine are arts intertwined with sciences that allow to broaden the mindset and approach of healthcare professionals. helping them to produce better care and more well-being.

Aim of this series is to collect "person-centered" contributions, as only a multidisciplinary and collaborative team can meet the challenge of combining the multiple aspects of human health, as well as the health of our planet, and of all the creatures that live on it, in a common effort to stop or reverse the enormous damage committed by humans during our anthropocentric era: a new paradigm of healthcare, education and learning to create a sustainable health system.

Gabriela-Paula Florea

Metacognition and Medical Humanities in Medical Education

The Missing Link in Medical Thinking

Springer

Gabriela-Paula Florea
Doctoral School of Philosophy
University of Bucharest
Bucharest, Romania

ISSN 2731-3247 ISSN 2731-3255 (electronic)
New Paradigms in Healthcare
ISBN 978-3-032-01069-8 ISBN 978-3-032-01070-4 (eBook)
https://doi.org/10.1007/978-3-032-01070-4

This Springer imprint is published by the registered company Springer Nature Switzerland AG
The registered company address is: Gewerbestrasse 11, 6330 Cham, Switzerland

To my family, Your belief in me has been my greatest strength, and your endless support has paved the way. This book is a tribute to your enduring presence and unwavering endorsement.

Foreword by Dorith Shaham

As a medical educator who founded a Medical Humanities program nearly two decades ago, I found this book to be truly eye-opening. It offers a compelling exploration of the cognitive and emotional dimensions of the medical encounter and introduces metacognition as a powerful tool to enhance both patient and physician satisfaction—and ultimately, health outcomes. Another key theme of the book is the integration of medical humanities as a means of strengthening the physician–patient relationship by fostering humanistic values and cultivating essential interpersonal skills—including critical thinking and empathic communication—through engagement with philosophy, literature, and the arts. By applying analytic philosophy to foundational concepts and practices in medicine, this book offers not only deep insights but also practical strategies for anyone engaged in the practice or teaching of medicine and medical humanities.

Hadassah Medical Center and Faculty of Medicine
Hebrew University of Jerusalem
Jerusalem, Israel

Dorith Shaham, M.D.

Foreword by Jonathan McFarland

I thank the author for this beautiful and brilliant book that captures both the intellectual spirit and emotional soul of the series New Paradigms in Healthcare. This is no surprise. I know the author and the book truly represents the author's determination and relentless hard work. The book is novel bringing something truly "new", which is no mean feat but perfectly captures the uniqueness of the author who is both a medical doctor and a philosopher. I am reminded of Galen of Pergamon, the great second-century Roman and Greek physician, who wrote "philosophy is necessary for physicians, it is clear that whoever is a physician must be altogether a philosopher." The author has brilliantly transferred the spirit of Galen to the needs of twenty-first-century health care. Her vision, as a doctor and a philosopher, is ideal for the troubled times we are living through. In a way, it reflects something I have always believed to be disconcerting; doctors and healthcare professionals have little time to reflect on their work, to think about why they do things, indeed, to reflect on, and think about their own thinking.

This is, of course, one of the missing links of twenty-first-century medicine and health care. For this reason alone, this book should be read by everyone who cares about the future of health care. Everyone.

Jonathan McFarland

Autonomous University of Madrid
Madrid, Spain

Pompeu Fabra University
Barcelona, Spain

The Doctor as a Humanist
Palma, Spain

Foreword

Metacognition and Medical Humanities in Medical Education: The Missing Link in Medical Thinking by Dr. Gabriela-Paula Florea offers a novel approach to a new groundbreaking topic in the philosophy and practice of medicine. A certified medical doctor and PhD in Philosophy, Dr. Florea brings to bear her combined expertise to this cutting-edge research at the cross-road of medical humanities, metacognition and medical thinking. As such, this original book grew out from her PhD dissertation that she defended at the University of Bucharest, Romania. Since the topic is brand new, there are only a handful of books discussing the issues of medical humanities. And for sure Florea's Dissertation and its present heir have been an absolute original novelty in her native Romania. The book explores the integration of metacognition and medical humanities in medical education and practice. Florea argues that modern medicine has experienced a divide between hard sciences and humanities, leading to a crisis in the quality of patient care. The book aims to reconcile these elements by emphasising the importance of cognitive awareness, compassionate interaction and metacognitive skills in medical practice.

The book firstly examines the historical tension between hard sciences and the humanities in medicine, highlighting in the process the increasing reliance on technology and the decline of humanistic values in patient care. Consequently, the book argues that one remedy to this drawback consists in taking a metacognition stance in medical humanities which can bridge this gap.

Part I of the book, "On Sense and Sensibility in Medicine", discusses gaps in understanding the doctor-patient relationship. The way Dr. Florea chooses to build the arguments is through criticising the dichotomy between paternalistic-authoritarian and humanistic-empathetic approaches. She introduces the concept of cognitive knowledge gaps in medical care.

In Part II, "The Doctor's and Patient's Extended Minds", Dr. Florea explores how cognitive processes influence the doctor-patient relationship. She analyses the placebo effect as evidence of the patient's extended mind, and suggests that patient cognition extends into the physician's thought process, impacting the outcomes.

Part III, "Metacognition and Medicine", defines metacognition and its relevance to medical decision-making; then the author examines the physiological and psychological effects of metacognitive processing in healthcare, and she discusses the role of intuition, socially shared metacognition and uncertainty in medicine.

Finally, in Part IV, "Conclusion: Medical Humanities and Metacognition as Missing Links", Dr. Florea argues that medical education must integrate metacognitive skills to improve patient outcomes and physician well-being. She highlights the necessity of a humanistic approach in conservative medical systems, and suggests that a shift in mindset, rather than just a paradigm shift, is essential to address the current crisis in healthcare.

The central argument of the whole book is articulated around the concept that metacognition—the ability to reflect on one's own thinking—and medical humanities should be fundamental aspects of medical education and practice. This approach can mitigate the dehumanisation of medicine by fostering better communication, empathy and cognitive adaptability among healthcare professionals.

Aristotle was one of the first important philosophers, if not the very first, who taught us that when people purposefully and conscientiously reflect on what they are doing, they would end up doing their things better. And this is why he invented/discovered formal logic. Metacognition, which amongst other things, means reflecting upon one's own practice in order to make it better or more efficient, is taken to the fullest and the highest level in Aristotle's study of valid reasoning. Now, if we extract a methodological lesson from all this, we can generalise and buy into the view that whenever we reach a critical point in making a practice better, one has to take the metacognitive stance. This is what Dr. Florea has undertaken in her wonderful and very timely research. She tells us that the landscape of modern medicine is continually evolving, shaped by the relentless pace of scientific discovery and the deepening understanding of the human condition. Amidst this dynamic environment, the interaction between healthcare providers and patients emerges as a pivotal arena, one that not only influences therapeutic outcomes but also defines the essence of medical practice.

Gabriela Florea's book has many virtues. Chief amongst those is that her research is devoted to this very new and groundbreaking topic which is medical humanities. The essence of the research is a multifaceted exploration of these "uncharted territories of the mental dimensions that underpin the doctor-patient relationship. It aims to explore the subtle yet profound ways in which metacognition (…) and the different facets of medical humanities can transform this relationship, enhancing both clinical judgment and patient care."

Gabriela Florea also shows why, and especially how, this topic which pertains to the medical sciences is also of genuine philosophical importance and interest. Moreover, she gives an answer to the rather sceptical question: what medical doctors could find out and learn from people who aim at philosophical clarifications and explanations? And indeed, Gabriela Florea is quick to point out that "at the core of this inquiry lies a fundamental question: How can the integration of metacognitive strategies and insights from medical humanities bridge the knowledge gap in understanding the mental dimension of the doctor-patient interaction?"

What is the practical value of this research, which from this perspective lies at the intersection of philosophy of medicine and applied/practical philosophy? In

Gabriela Florea's own words: „Through this approach, the dissertation aims to construct a more nuanced framework for patient care, one that transcends the traditional biomedical model by incorporating the complexities of human thought, experience and the biological interplay between medical condition and metacognition."

The book is very complex and thorough, exploring a comprehensive review of relevant literature, qualitative analyses of patient and healthcare provider experiences. But what only someone like Dr. Florea, with a solid background knowledge in philosophy, can bring to the debate, and indeed does bring to the discussion, is a theoretical exploration of concepts from contemporary domains of philosophy which are relevant to this topic. Dr. Florea makes use of some of the newest powerful and innovative philosophical theories coming from philosophical logic, philosophy of language and mostly philosophy of mind, viz. Kit Fine's semantic relationism, and the integrated approach of 4Es in mind and cognition: embodied, embedded, enactive and extended mind and cognition, which is a relatively young and thriving field of interdisciplinary research. Roughly, it assumes that cognition is shaped and structured by dynamic interactions between the brain, body and both the physical and social environments.

Now, to give you a rough sketch of this philosophical background in order to appreciate the importance of Gabriela Florea's contribution to developing a solid philosophical foundation for medical humanities suffices to point out that Kit Fine's semantic relationist approach to meaning is deepening the conception about how the meanings of propositions depend not only on the semantic features and roles of each separate meaningful unit in a complex but also on the relations that those units hold to each other; Fine holds that semantic relations that have to be added to the assigned intrinsic values in our semantic theory, especially the relation which he calls "coordination", can do much of the work of senses.

The programme defends *referentialism* in philosophy of language. Semantic relationism gives a finer-grained definition of compositionality, which is an essential feature for understanding the systematicity and productivity of the mind and the language. I cannot go into any technical detail here. Suffices to say that this semantic and philosophical discussion brings along a new relational view of language and mind. Now, after this concise presentation of Kit Fine's thoughts on meaning, the extension of this semantic relationist outlook to the patient-physician relationship is quite natural and obvious according to Dr. Florea. And indeed, she explores this important analogy. The medical strategy and behaviour would greatly improve if thought along the lines of this sort of relationism.

But it is less obvious how to use the extended mind view in such a way that inserting metacognition into the patient-physician relationships would give philosophical substance to the medical humanities. And this is precisely what Florea does which, to my opinion, is the most important philosophical feature of her research. Florea's idea is that a medical doctor is, or better acts, as the extended mind of the patient. This in itself is a major change of the mind set when it comes to the understating of the physician-patient relationship (especially in the Romanian context!).

But what is this 4Es (extended/embodied/embedded/enactive) mind approach about? Embodied Cognition (as a general umbrella) is a complex interdisciplinary research programme based on work in psychology, neuroscience, ethology, philosophy, linguistics, robotics and artificial intelligence. Traditional cognitive science also draws on these disciplines, and its telling feature is that mind is the medium of computation: mental processes are computational processes; the brain, *qua* computer, is the seat of cognition. But in contradistinction to this traditional reductionist vision, Embodied Cognition rejects or rephrases the computational stance of cognitive science, stressing instead upon the significance of an agent's physical body in cognitive abilities. The main unifying concept is that the body or the body's interactions with the environment constitute or contribute to cognition. Mental processes are not, or not only, computational processes. The brain is not a computer, or not the seat of cognition; cognition lies at the intersection of mind and body and external factors in the environment.

To wrap up, the book is a valuable contribution to the ongoing debate on how to improve both medical practice and education. To achieve those desiderata, it goes into a deeper understanding of the complex doctor-patient relationship, emphasising the roles of cognition. Through the analysis of these dimensions of the medical humanities and the metacognitive strategies, Dr. Florea gives valuable insights that could lead to more humane, effective and compassionate medical care in modern medicine.

Dr. Gabriela Florea's book presents an interdisciplinary perspective, integrating philosophy, neuroscience and medical education. It suggests that recognising and developing metacognitive skills through medical humanities programmes can help rehumanise modern medicine and improve both patient care and physician wellbeing. As such, the book is a valuable addition to the field of philosophy of medicine that will be of real interest both to MDs interested in the metacognitive aspects and skills of their practice, and also to those scholars interested in medical thinking and applications of cognitive science and philosophy to the field of the philosophy of medicine.

Vice-president of the Romanian Academy Mircea Dumitru
University of Bucharest
Bucharest, Romania

Preface

This book, *Metacognition and Medical Humanities in Medical Education: The Missing Link in Medical Thinking*, is the culmination of my doctoral research undertaken at the University of Bucharest. As both a medical doctor and a philosopher, I have long been fascinated by the intersection between clinical reasoning and reflective thought, between scientific rigour and human experience. This work seeks to articulate and explore a critical yet under-examined question: what is lost when medicine neglects the metacognitive and humanistic dimensions of its practice?

In contemporary medical education, the dominance of the biomedical model and evidence-based methodologies has brought undeniable advances. Yet, this same dominance has contributed to a disconnection from the patient's experiential world: physicians, who are trained to diagnose with precision, are rarely encouraged to reflect on their own thinking, on the structure and limits of their knowledge or on the moral and emotional dimensions of the doctor–patient relationship. This book argues that we need more than technical training—we need metacognitive awareness, philosophical insight and humane responsiveness.

This research proposes that metacognition—understood as the capacity to reflect upon and regulate one's own cognitive processes—together with insights from the medical humanities, can become a powerful tool for improving not only clinical outcomes but also the lived experiences of both patients and healthcare providers. By reframing the doctor–patient interaction through this dual lens, we can cultivate deeper empathy, better communication and greater professional self-awareness.

The intended audience includes medical educators, practising physicians, students in medicine and philosophy, researchers interested in the intersections of cognitive science, ethics and the medical humanities, as well as members of the general public who are curious about the human dimension of healthcare. This book is also for those who believe, as I do, that the most effective medicine arises from the integration of rigorous knowledge with the capacity for critical self-reflection and compassion.

While this book is grounded in the Romanian context in which the original research was conducted, the issues it addresses are universal. The challenges of fragmentation, depersonalisation and burnout in medicine transcend national borders. It is my hope that this work contributes to an emerging international dialogue on how best to rehumanise medicine—not by turning away from science but by integrating it more deeply with reflection, empathy and philosophical insight.

I am grateful to Springer Nature for offering this book a wider platform, and to the many scholars, mentors and colleagues who have helped shape the ideas contained within. I now offer them to the reader, in the spirit of inquiry, collaboration and care.

Bucharest, Romania
May 2025

Gabriela-Paula Florea

Competing Interests

The author has no conflicts of interest to declare relevant to this book's content.

Acknowledgements

First and foremost, I would like to express my heartfelt gratitude to my advisor, Professor Mircea Dumitru whose constant support, expertise, insightful guidance and encouragement have been invaluable in my research and in completing this book.

I am also deeply grateful to Prof. Dorith Shaham. Her mentorship and insight have significantly contributed to my professional development and shaped my research. Her guidance, particularly in medical humanities, has been instrumental.

Pivotal in my research process were the insightful meetings with the distinguished teaching staff from the Medical Education Centre, Hadassah Medical School, at the Hebrew University of Jerusalem during my research internship in 2019 under the supervision of Prof. Dorith Shaham. To all of them, I express my sincere and deepest gratitude and respect for their openness in sharing their experience in developing the first medical humanities programme in Israel, Adam U'Refuah (the human being and medicine), as well as for allowing me to participate at the End of Life and Palliative Care module.

I would also like to extend my sincere thanks to my co-editor, Prof. Viorel Cernica, Faculty of Philosophy at the University of Bucharest, and co-authors, Prof. Daniela Dumitru and Lecturer Mihaela Minciu, Department of Teacher Training at the Bucharest Academy of Economic Studies, for their valuable contributions to the volumes and chapters we published together.

I am thankful to my doctoral programme committee members, Prof. Laurentiu Staicu, Prof. Viorel Vizureanu and Prof. Gheorghe Ştefanov, whose constructive feedback and insightful suggestions greatly enhanced the quality of this work and its outcome.

I am deeply thankful to Prof. Margareta Fleşner for introducing me to the field of analytic philosophy. Her guidance shaped my academic pathway.

I also express my heartfelt appreciation to Michael McGrath for his invaluable insights into the scientific fluency of my arguments, which enriched the depth and quality of this research.

I am indebted to esteemed Romanian scholars for their involvement in the medical humanities programmes we developed at the University of Bucharest and the

University of Medicine and Pharmacy "Carol Davila" Bucharest. Their stimulating discussions and contributions to the multidimensional doctor-patient relationship have significantly enriched my research experience. Among them are Professors Viorel Jinga, Bogdan Ovidiu Popescu, Emil Toescu, Liviu Lucaci; Associate Professors Sorin Costreie, Ştefan Busnatu, Emanuel Socaciu, Constantin Vică; Senior Lecturers Anamaria Neagu, Dana Popescu-Spineni and Raluca Tatar; and PhD candidates Ioan Mirea and Ioana Alexandra Răduca.

For the international collaborative projects, I would also like to express my gratitude to esteemed Professors Marianna Karamanou and Jonathan McFarland for co-organising the first CIVIS European Summer School on Medical Humanities, Inclusive Approaches to The Medical Humanities, hosted by the National and Kapodistrian University of Athens in May 2022, and all others involved. Moreover, I would like to express my deepest gratitude to Prof. McFarland for allowing me to share my knowledge on metacognition in medicine and medical education in all the projects committed to "putting heart and soul back into medicine" through The Doctor as a Humanist organisation. My most profound appreciation also goes to Lexi Nguyen and Faith Chadwick, founders of the Students for Health Humanities Association. They made possible the connection with numerous esteemed professors of health humanities from US universities, such as Lise Saffran (College of Health Sciences, University of Missouri, USA), Dr. Kamna Balhara (Johns Hopkins Medicine, Hopkins Krieger School of Arts and Science, USA) and Amanda M. Caleb (Geisinger Commonwealth School of Medicine, Scranton, Pennsylvania, USA), without whom programmes developed in the Romanian academic field would not have been so rich and insightful.

I gratefully acknowledge the support of the Centre of Innovation and e-Health at the University of Medicine and Pharmacy "Carol Davila" Bucharest, coordinated by Associate Prof. Ştefan Busnatu, for their support in developing medical humanities programmes through projects financed through CNFIS-FDI-2023-F-0709--FUTUREMED and CNFIS-FDI-2022-0594-INOPRACT.

I would like to express my gratitude to all teaching staff from the Faculty of Philosophy at the University of Bucharest for their input, especially to Bianca Savu, for her constructive observations on my first writings on analytical philosophy and her enduring presence during my first steps in this journey. Special thanks to all my colleagues from the Doctoral School of Philosophy for the insightful discussions throughout these years. Extended thanks to all healthcare students and professionals who have participated in our medical and health humanities programmes and shared their experiences in the medical education and healthcare system, which have been valuable for my research work.

A big thank you to the administrative staff of the Faculty of Philosophy, including Ecaterina Matei, Viviana and Lilian Ciachir, for their assistance with logistics and paperwork, without whom this research work would not have seen the light of day.

I wish to extend my deepest thanks to my family for their endless support and encouragement. To my parents, Liana-Rodica and Adrian, for their love and belief in me, my sister Mihaela and her family, and other family members who are too numerous to mention here. Also, to my friends, Ana Gubrei, Daniela Hudelcu, Yanki Shapira, Alina Simion, Anamaria Neagu, Elena Bădiulescu and Bogdan Nicolaide, for their constant encouragement and for always being there when I needed them.

Last but not least, I wish to thank my patients, without whom the need and purpose of this endeavour would not have had significance, and Dr. John Upledger for having inspired me to reach the concept of metacognitive processes. Through his teachings on CranioSacral Therapy and SomatoEmotional Release®, Dr. Upledger's method is an essential tool in my practice in supporting patients in connecting their minds and bodies. Also, I show my appreciation to all Upledger Institute International professors who shared their knowledge and experience with me.

In the end, I am profoundly grateful to everyone who has, directly or indirectly, been part of this journey.

Contents

About the Author

Gabriela-Paula Florea is a pioneering scholar in metacognition and medical humanities in medical education. Born in Romania, she defended her PhD thesis, *Transforming Medical Practice: Metacognition in Medical Education*, at the University of Bucharest on July 8, 2024, under the guidance of Professor Mircea Dumitru. Her thesis is groundbreaking as the first to explore metacognition in the doctor-patient relationship globally and in medical humanities in Romania.

She holds a bachelor's degree in general medicine from "Carol Davila" University of Medicine and Pharmacy and advanced certification in CranioSacral therapy from the Upledger Institute International. She has worked as a Medical Humanities Program Coordinator, lecturer, Public Health Resident Physician at Craiova County Emergency Clinical Hospital and Pedagogical Recovery Therapist for individuals with autism spectrum disorders.

Her academic contributions include innovative research on metacognition in medicine and the transformation of medical practice in post-Communist Romania. She has organised workshops and courses integrating critical thinking and metacognitive strategies into medical education and practice, and presented her work at international conferences on the philosophy of medicine and medical humanities.

Her editorial work includes co-editing volumes on contemporary philosophical research and contributing to notable publications such as *Developing the Intuitive Executive* (CRC Press) and *Brain, Decision Making and Mental Health* (Springer). Her dedication to advancing medical education through humanistic and metacognitive approaches has established her as a leader in the field.

Abbreviations

dACC	Dorsal anterior cingulate cortex
AD	Anno Domini
AP	Attending physician
BC	Before Christ
BMM	Biomedical model
BPS	Bio-psycho-social
BPSM	Bio-psycho-social model
CAS	Cognitive attentional syndrome
CBT	Cognitive behavioural therapy
COVID	Coronavirus disease
CPGS	Chronic Pain Grade Scale
DNA	Deoxyribonucleic acid
EBM	Evidence-based medicine
EM	Extended mind
EMT	Extended mind theory
EU	European Union
GAD	Generalised anxiety disorder
GDP	Gross domestic product
GST	General systems theory
HA	Health anxiety
HPA	Hypothalamic-pituitary-adrenal
IQ	Intelligence quotient
MCQ-HA	Metacognitions Questionnaire-Health Anxiety
MCT	Metacognitive therapy
ME	Metacognitive experiences
MF	Metacognitive feelings
MK	Metacognitive knowledge
MR	Metacognitive regulation
NBM	Narrative-based medicine
OCD	Obsessive-compulsive disorder
PAP	Physician-as-patient

PCM	Patient-centred medicine
PM	Personalised medicine
PNEI	Psycho-neuro-endocrine-immunology
PTSD	Post-traumatic stress disorder
RDBPC	Randomised double-blind placebo-controlled (clinical trial)
SDM	Shared decision-making
SHAI	Short Health Anxiety Inventory
SMM	Shared mental model
SSM	Socially shared metacognition
TM	Translational medicine
VBM	Value-based medicine

List of Figures

List of Tables

Chapter 1
Introduction

The title of this book captures two major domains—medical education and practice—bridged by two complex fields—metacognition and medical humanities as key concepts that may address the quality-of-care crisis in modern medicine.

Philosophy has been debating medical education and practice as well as the humanities for the past centuries with important figures such as Sir William Osler [1], Edmund Pellegrino [2–5] and James Marcum [6–9] bringing substance to what has appeared to be a never-ending debate regarding the role of the humanities within the art of medicine. Kazem Sadegh-Zadeh [10] has even been able to bring the discussion to the level of decision-making processes with his logical and philosophical underpinnings that influence clinical thinking and the overall interaction between doctors and patients. Whilst these debates date back to the early nineteenth century, a worldwide consensus about the Science-Humanity interplay in medical practice seems far from over.

Metacognition, though, is rarely discussed in medicine. It is notably used tangentially in medical education via Problem-Based Learning (PBL) approaches [11–14] and metaemotions [15]. Although, at first glance, metacognition and medical humanities seem to have nothing in common, this book not only justifies their interdependency but also offers a novel insight into how their reliance on each other may bridge knowledge gaps in understanding the root cause of the dehumanisation of medical practice, in an expanding high-tech and low-touch modern medicine.

1.1 Did Science and Humanity Divorce?

From the first decades of philosophical debates on medicine, it appears that medical practice underwent a divorce between Science and its longstanding and dependent relationship with Humanity. Medicine had to choose between the old-fashioned

G.-P. Florea, *Metacognition and Medical Humanities in Medical Education*, New Paradigms in Healthcare, https://doi.org/10.1007/978-3-032-01070-4_1

humanities in favour of the fashionable, new and sparkling sciences as if they could not be part of the same family. This now leaves us in this brand-new House of Medicine, where patients are at the mercy of a false dilemma in which practitioners must choose between Science and Humanity.

From the research this book presents, it is not about one or the other but about the lost Humanity, even in the philosophical discourse that should regard medical professionals' well-being as much as the patients and their family and friends. From this allegoric standpoint, it feels as if the physician, the child of these two alternative couples (Medicine-Science or Medicine-Humanity), must choose one to spend their time with. Similar to most examples, the child is the most affected, since the "adults" in this house (Medicine as a complex multilayered and vital domain) have more power and more knowledge regarding life and what is correct for the "family." So, the child always suffers the most. The subtext of this dispute between the "adults of the family"—Science and Humanity—even impacts the last lost child of medicine, namely, the medical professionals. This is how the problem between Science and Humanity controls the dynamic between their children (medical professionals and patients) in which their families and friends are no exception.

Throughout this era of disputes, philosophy has offered the necessary and rich field of debates for reconciliation, which has reached maturity. Now is the time to propose clear actions regarding the future of this marriage between two strong-headed, co-dependent strengths, Science and Humanity, and their children (medical professionals and patients), who all must share the same house, Medicine. In order to prosper they must also find peace and harmony, with the wise and gentle Humanity complementing the pragmatic solution-oriented Science for they are not enemies but companions sharing the same objective.

1.2 The Science's Pragmatism and the Humanity's Wisdom

Ever since the era of Asklepios, the House of Medicine has had a more spiritual foundation, since whenever a person was suffering from what we now would call a "physiological dysfunction" or medical condition, it was divine-sent, and Asklepios, the God, was responsible for treating the ill [16, 17]. Later, this divine paradigm changed, with Hippocrates stating the case for a medicine based on observation and logic, which Galen raised to another level of understanding of the human body by reducing it to its parts, and hence the inception of the next paradigm shift: reductionism [18, 19].

In the seventeenth century, Descartes brought the mind-body dualism into the discussion, further reducing the body to its parts, a vision that went hand-in-hand with the Newtonian mechanical view applied to the understanding of the body [20–24]. At the beginning of the nineteenth century, Claude Bernard emphasised the importance of understanding the body's internal environment and how various body parts contribute to homeostasis [25]. In the nineteenth and twentieth centuries with the rise of biology, chemistry and molecular biology, access to the smallest body parts was made possible: discovering cellular and molecular parts of human genetics. The discovery of the structure of DNA [26] and its function contributed to the research of epigenetics, which proved how the environment could influence gene expression and manifestation leading to the critical hypothesis that the environment can influence body changes [27]. All these microscopic discoveries drove the development of personalised and precision medicine by treating patients according to their unique genetic makeup [28]. Moreover, the psycho-neuro-endocrine-immunology field of research fully understood the importance of the mind-body-environment interconnection and its impact on human health and disease [29].

Until the discovery of the microscope, the human body was studied macroscopically through open-eye observations, and only in the last 500 years or so have we been able to explore the smallest parts of the human body, down to its subatomic chemical components. These advancements have been as significant for understanding the anatomy and physiology of the human body as exploring outer space has been for understanding the universe. Just as new inventions have allowed us to venture into the cosmos, they have also enabled us to journey into our "inner space," transforming medicine's understanding of human anatomy, biology and the chemical and physical laws governing life. Great discoveries have been made possible by great inventions. Therefore, it is unfair to blame technology or its scientific instruments for justifying medicine's disregard of humanity. However, the same technological power that allows us to reach otherwise inaccessible territories in outer space may tempt us to prioritise that over the humanity that defines us. This visible tension underscores the need to balance scientific advancement with preserving the human essence in medicine.

Therefore, technology's contribution to this *zooming in* and *out* of the human body has greatly contributed to modern medical epistemology. Have we *zoomed in* enough to understand all the mysteries of the human body? No. But we have reached a strong enough understanding of it to act accordingly when treating a patient. Have we *zoomed out* enough to comprehend the interplay between the human body and the environment, including nature and social interactions? Perhaps, but there are still many things left to discover. However, we do have an important body of information to acknowledge the impact that the outer setting from the surrounding physical space, and the unique social relationship between the doctor and the patient has on the clinical outcome. The impact of these different settings is so important that clinicians have reached historical levels of stress and frustration in their daily practice and burnout has a plague-like prevalence.

1.3 Questions and Objectives

Thus, we have reached one of the core problems of modern medicine: medical professionals find it difficult to cope with the enormous workload in a conveyor-belt interaction with patients, influenced by the restraints of the medical system. The time with one patient is often limited to 10 min, during which the doctor has to acquire the information needed to make a correct diagnosis and propose treatment plans as well as discussing them with the patient to reach a shared decision and create a symmetrical rapport whilst remaining faithful to their credo.

If this is how things are happening at a grassroots level, at the meta-level, it is far more complicated. We are talking about layers of understanding human conditions in a clinical context and how they address the patients' needs so that medical professionals can place the patient at the centre whilst offering the best expert knowledge for the optimal healthcare outcome within extreme time-limits. In this respect, the philosophical debate argues that modern medicine rarely accomplishes this ideal, since medical professionals rely more on technological advancement than listening to the patient, amongst other issues.

At an even deeper conceptual level, the discussion leaps towards the biomedical (or reductionist-paternalistic) and biopsychosocial (or holistic-humanistic) as possible options for treating patients. Is one approach better than the other? Should patients be reduced to their parts, or should they be acknowledged holistically, within the mind-body-environment?

Starting from these current philosophical themes, this book makes a thorough examination of the underlying causes, identifying knowledge gaps and accurately understanding the level that medicine has reached to comprehend that the answers reside, de facto, from the latest discoveries: (1) the relationship between the mind and the body is currently explained by psycho-neuro-endocrine-immunology and precision or personalised medicine, and (2) the results found from the research on the placebo phenomenon with its neurobiological changes describe the underlying mechanism behind the doctor-patient relationship.

The book's objectives consist of separating the layers of this problem. Consequently, the identified layers involve the following:

1. Medical epistemology and paradigm shifts throughout the history of medicine, answering the question, "What is science telling us today about the human body, the mind and its relationship with the environment? A follow-up question might be: "Should doctors treat patients mechanically or holistically?"
2. Another layer concerns cognition and metacognition, cognitive and metacognitive processes that develop in the doctor-patient relationship. How relevant are they in the relationship's economy? Considering the purpose of this unique social interaction, what are the implications on an individual and relationship level?
3. The third layer regards education, which is the core from which true reforms in shaping the understanding of knowledge as the key to updating the current default mechanical and reductionist view of medicine. Can medical education bring the current scientific mind-body enviromental (holistic) view of medicine into clinical practice?

The aim is to connect these complex layers and highlight the knowledge gaps revealed by the *bench to bedside* conceptual contamination in understanding the doctor-patient relationship and how it shapes it in the following ways:

- The unique social status of the medical encounter and the outdated or conservative mentality in not accepting new key findings of the human body and its relationship with the environment; adding to this the extended mind theory that can explain how the patient relies on the physician's mind, thus extending into their world
- The metacognitive mind power that humans have, especially explicit metacognition, has been under-explored in research regarding its role for medical professionals and patients and its impact on patients' outcomes and medical professional well-being

1.4 The Central Argument and the Methodological Approach

This book pursues the path to link these knowledge gaps with medical humanities programmes that, until empirical research proves the opposite, can theoretically foster and develop the metacognitive awareness skill, which may be a solution to the quality-of-care crisis that can represent the source and the resource to rehumanise modern medicine.

Within an interdisciplinary framework, this book adopts an analytic philosophical approach through a multifaceted research methodology, drawing upon a comprehensive literature review, qualitative analyses of patient and healthcare provider experiences, and a theoretical exploration through challenging thought experiments. Therefore, it brings Kit Fine's semantic relationism theory [30] to analyse the significance of the healthcare provider and the patient's internal features within their binomial rapport. Moreover, in the context of how the patient may think about their own thinking when ill, this book builds on John Flavell's [31] theory on developmental psychology regarding metacognitive thinking, highlighting the possibility of patients with chronic diseases using problem-solving methods that employ metacognitive processes to illustrate their impact on both patients and healthcare professionals at biological and cognitive levels. Other essential derivates of metacognition regard the socially shared metacognition and intuition in medical practice, underscoring their critical role in addressing uncertainties. Moreover, the book brings forward an argument that links Andy Clark and David Chalmers' extended mind theory [32] with the placebo effect and response [33]. In addition, it offers a case study to examine the possibility of a shift from a paternalistic-based system to a relationship-centred approach in conservative medical systems to justify, once more, how medical humanities and metacognitive awareness are the missing links of modern medicine.

Throughout the debates and studies on the doctor-patient relationship, most have focussed primarily on either the perspective of medical professionals or on patients. Unlike approaches that treat these perspectives separately, this book brings them into conversation with each other. It looks closely at each side on its own, but also at how they interact, because in any real relationship, each part shapes and is shaped by the other.

It is a long-standing challenge that philosophers and scientists often find collaboration difficult, not due to lack of interest, but because of the divergent languages and conceptual frameworks inherent to their disciplines. In an effort to bridge this divide, the style of writing adopted in this work consciously balances philosophical rigour with accessibility, making space for engagement from clinicians, scholars in the humanities, and an informed general readership. Facilitating productive exchanges between theoretical and clinical domains is not merely desirable—it is imperative if we are to address persistent shortcomings in healthcare practice. To maintain clarity and coherence, and to avoid excessive terminological distinction, the terms "medical humanities" and "health humanities" are treated synonymously throughout.

1.5 The Roadmap of the Science-Humanity Divorce to Reconciliation

This book accomplishes the task of linking the identified knowledge gaps with medical humanities programmes as a means to develop and/or foster the meta-cognitive awareness skill; a solution to the quality-of-care crisis that may possibly represent the source and the resource to rehumanise modern medicine through the following four parts:

Part I, *On Sense and Sensibility*, aims to capture the two contrasting qualities of the human mind and behaviour and emotions that are always present in clinical practice. As in Jane Austen's novel, the central theme of this part revolves around the philosophical perspectives involved. In this case, it rationalises what scientific achievements have brought to medicine and how they can be transposed into clinical practice without altering Humanity. The key to balancing the sense of medical science with the sensibility of those involved in practising medicine highlights the importance of finding this balance between the *hard sciences* and the *soft feelings* embedded in interpersonal and professional relationships.

When discussing sense in medicine, it is necessary to change from the paradigm shift debate to a mentality shift debate, since the modern paradigm shift in medicine (reductionist medicine to whole medicine) has already started. Thus, it is time to focus on how scientific changes have enhanced the understanding of the human body, reaching a holistic view, and how this leap should be aligned with or in tune with how medical education shapes future doctors: not in the reductionist paradigm but the holistic one.

Part II, *On the Doctors and Patients' Extended Minds*, brings arguments in favour of the interconnectedness between patients' and doctors' cognitive processes manifested within their relationship, claiming that the patient's mind is extended to the mind of the physician. The explanations of the placebo phenomenon and the neurobiological changes behind the doctor-patient relationship come as an endorsement of the patient's extended mind.

Part III, *On Metacognition And Medicine*, brings metacognition into medical play, stating that metacognitive awareness plays a pivotal role for both patients and medical practitioners, impacting the patient's outcomes and the practitioner's mental well-being. The patient's response to a negative diagnosis is discussed through first- and second-order mental processing and highlights the physiological changes that can occur in receiving the diagnosis and, further, how they can face the future in a problem-solving mental attitude. This chapter also brings two derivates of metacognitive thinking—socially shared metacognition and intuition—as relevant to possible volatile, uncertain, complex or ambiguous situations that can occur in medical practice.

Part IV, *Medical Humanities and Metacognition: Modern Medicine's Missing Links*, concludes the book by bringing together all the central elements of the book's core statement, showcasing that medicine without acknowledging the metacognitive thinking role will only deepen the quality-of-care crisis, whilst metacognition in medicine without medical humanities is impossible, since this pervasive skill cannot be fostered without the humanistic disciplines applied in medical education and practice.

Whilst these four parts stand by themselves, presenting independently strong claims, they share one central issue that is found repeatedly in most of the modern philosophical debates on medicine, namely, the association between (1) the biomedical model that guides medical professionals, with reductionism and paternalism, and (2) the biopsychosocial model that guides physician, with holism and humanism. Each chapter thus presents independent arguments that contrast this view by stating that a biomedical-guided practitioner, considered to adhere to paternalism automatically, does not necessarily imply detached concern and presenting themselves as authoritarians, as much as the biopsychosocial-guided practitioner does not necessarily imply manifesting empathetic care. However, the answer to this issue resides in the importance of being aware of the belief system and the needs of both patients and medical professionals. They may clash sometimes, but the differences must always be accepted and respected. Consequently, that "doctors should adopt" an empathetic concern when approaching a patient should be changed to that "doctors should adapt" to each patient's belief system to respond to their specific needs that stem from this understanding. Therefore, the need for metacognitive awareness skills (the missing link in medical education) developed through medical humanities programmes should be mandatory.

1.6 Contribution to Reconciliation

This interdisciplinary book brings a novelty to the doctor-patient relationship; the metacognitive level, which has never been previously addressed in the specialised literature. Moreover, the theoretical proof between medical humanities programmes and metacognitive awareness in medical education and continuous professional development (CPD) programmes is another stepping-stone to making enhanced medical care that impacts all the involved actors. By examining these dimensions within the context of metacognitive strategies through medical humanities programmes, this pioneering theoretical research offers valuable insights that could lead to innovative future research for more effective and healthier approaches to medical care in a "high-tech" and "low-touch" modern medicine.

If the duel between Humanity and Science persists, it is destined to end in a draw, for the forces driving them—wisdom and knowledge—are measured by the same unit: power. Furthermore, the power each wields is perfectly balanced, with neither overcoming the other. The primary barrier to resolving this confrontation and breaking the tension within the House of Medicine lies in the mindset of its practitioners. However, what appears to be a vicious circle can be transformed into a virtuous one, provided Education assumes the role of the impartial referee.

References

1. Osler W (1919) The old humanities and the new science. BMJ 2:1–7
2. Pellegrino ED, Thomasma DC (1993) The virtues in medical practice. Oxford University Press, New York
3. Pellegrino E (2005) The "telos" of medicine and the good of the patient. In: Clinical Bioethics, pp 21–32
4. Pellegrino ED (1998) What the philosophy of medicine is. Theor Med Bioeth 19:315–336
5. Pellegrino ED (1986) Philosophy of medicine: towards a definition. J Med Philos 11:9–16
6. Marcum JA (2008) An introductory philosophy of medicine: humanizing modern medicine. Philos Med. https://doi.org/10.1007/978-1-4020-6797-6
7. Marcum JA (2021) P7 medicine: humanizing systems medicine. Teorema 40:215–231
8. Marcum JA (2008) Reflections on humanizing biomedicine. Perspect Biol Med 51:392–405
9. Marcum JA (2017) The Bloomsbury companion to contemporary philosophy of medicine. Bloomsbury Academic, London
10. Sadegh-Zadeh K (2015) Handbook of analytic philosophy of medicine. Springer, Dordrecht. https://doi.org/10.1007/978-94-017-9579-1
11. Güner P, Erbay HN (2021) Metacognitive skills and problem-solving. Int J Res Educ Sci 7:715–734
12. Barrows HS (1996) Problem-based learning in medicine and beyond: a brief overview. New Dir Teach Learn 1996:3–12
13. Chan ZCY (2017) A qualitative study on using concept maps in problem-based learning. Nurse Educ Pract 24:70–76
14. Tseng F-Y, Shieh J-Y, Kao T-W, Wu C-C, Chu T-S, Chen Y-Y (2016) Developing and evaluating medical humanities problem-based learning classes facilitated by the teaching assistants majored in the Liberal arts: a longitudinal crossover study. Medicine 95(6):e2765. https://doi.org/10.1097/MD.0000000000002765
15. Dinsmore DL (2017) Examining the ontological and epistemic assumptions of research on metacognition, self-regulation and self-regulated learning. Educ Psychol (Lond) 37:1125–1153
16. Edelstein EJ, Edelstein L (1945) Asclepius: a collection and interpretation of the testimonies. Johns Hopkins Press. https://doi.org/10.2307/4342353
17. Curnow T (2012) The cult of Asclepius: its origins and early development. Bull John Rylands Univ Libr Manchester 89:67–83
18. Hippocrates (2015) The complete works of Hippocrates. Delphi Classics
19. Galen (1916) On the natural faculties. Harvard University Press, Cambridge, MA

20. Bottaccioli F (2014) La fine della grande illusione del riduzionismo in biologia e in medicina. In: Epistemologia, pp 5–21
21. Spencer D (2017) Narrative medicine. In: Solomon M, Simon JR, Kincaid H (eds) The Routledge companion to philosophy of medicine. Routledge, pp 372–382
22. O'Leary D (2021) Medicine's metaphysical morass: how confusion about dualism threatens public health. Synthese 199:1977–2005
23. Gold J (1985) Cartesian dualism and the current crisis in medicine—a plea for a philosophical approach: discussion paper. J R Soc Med 78:663–666
24. Duncan G (2000) Mind-body dualism and the biopsychosocial model of pain: what did Descartes really say? J Med Philos 25:485–513
25. Ramachandran VS (2012) Encyclopedia of human behavior, 2nd edn. Elsevier/Academic, London/Burlington
26. Watson JD, Crick FHC (1953) Molecular structure of nucleic acids: a structure for deoxyribose nucleic acid. Nature 171:737–738
27. Goldberg AD, Allis CD, Bernstein E (2007) Epigenetics: a landscape takes shape. Cell 128:635–638
28. Collins FS, Fink L (1995) The human genome project. Alcohol Health Res World 19:190–195
29. Kusnecov AW, Anisman H (2014) The Wiley-Blackwell handbook of psychoneuroimmunology, 1st edn. Wiley
30. Fine K (2007) Semantic relationism. Wiley-Blackwell, New York. https://doi.org/10.1002/9780470690826
31. Flavell JH (1979) Metacognition and cognitive monitoring. A new area of cognitive-developmental inquiry. Am Psychol 34:906–911
32. Clark A, Chalmers D (1998) The extended mind. Analysis. https://doi.org/10.1093/analys/58.1.7
33. Benedetti F (2011) The patient's brain: the neuroscience behind the doctor-patient relationship. Oxford University Press, Oxford

Part I
On Sense and Sensibility in Medicine

Chapter 2
Gaps in Understanding the Doctor-Patient Relationship

2.1 Are Paternalistic-Authoritarian and Humanistic-Empathetic Correlations True Axioms?

Doctor-patient types of interactions are generally classified as paternalistic, associated with biomedical, and humanistic with biopsychosocial models of medical practice [1]. This classification is globally accepted, but at the same time, there are many debates as to which should be applied in clinical practice [1–7]. Philosophers of medicine usually associate paternalism with a non-humanistic-oriented practice [1], where paternalism is mistaken for an authoritarian attitude. In the paternalistic approach, the doctor is a father figure who acts accordingly for the patient's benefit. At the same time, authoritarianism intrinsically implies domination, oppression and a coercive attitude [8], which opposes the Hippocratic oath, and goes against a genuine doctor's *modus operandi.*

According to Gérard Reach's definition, patient education in chronic care empowers the patient to make collaborative decisions with the healthcare provider [9] and, therefore, the link between patient autonomy and medical education leads to a paradox, a conflict between the patient's principle of autonomy and the physician's principle of beneficence [9, 10]. The most common example is when the patient is uneducated, they may have difficulties in understanding the information. It is also true that advocating patient autonomy is synonymous with respect, whilst disregarding it denotes a lack of respect. In this case, the medical professional may have to make some of the decisions, which may imply a paternalistic approach, and the paradox arises, since the patient's autonomy cannot be fully protected.

There should be a strong distinction between the paternalistic approach and doctor-centred medicine, since paternalism does not necessarily imply doctor-centeredness, whilst doctor-centeredness implies paternalism. The association between paternalistic and non-humanistic approaches may also be superficial and

G.-P. Florea, *Metacognition and Medical Humanities in Medical Education*, New Paradigms in Healthcare, https://doi.org/10.1007/978-3-032-01070-4_2

cognitively error leading. From my perspective, the classification has been made from an erroneously applied concept, namely, "patient-centeredness," as an opposing solution to "doctor-centeredness." I claim that both views have significant flaws that arise from ignoring the word "relationship" within the doctor-patient dyad.

2.1.1 The Doctor-Patient Dyad

Medical epistemology is the common ground that all medical practitioners share, no matter which side they take. What differs in their practice, though, is the humane aspect they wish, or not, to manifest. In a broad sense, in their rapport with the patients, doctors guide their practice based on different schools of thought, which unfold on three levels: conceptual, decision making, and relational. The first revolves around the concept of health and disease, the second is related to the parties they choose to be involved in the clinical decision-making process and the third is behaviouristic in the sense of how they choose to approach the patient at an interpersonal (relational) level.

The "ideological" system of practicing medicine is being embraced by medical practitioners according to their set of beliefs and depends on the doctor's degree of openness. The key factors are independent, but also coexist, are interrelated and work on overlapping plans that take place simultaneously: (1) the meaning physicians assume concerning the concept of disease reflected in their approach to the patient, (2) the adopted method when having to make decisions depends on how to approach the patient, personal or impersonal, and following from this, (3) the approach they choose in communicating with the patient based on the previous two plans. These layers that form the clinical act take place in the context of the doctor-patient relationship, thus being of significant importance when trying to define the doctor's blueprint for performing the clinical ritual. The proof that little importance has been given to the patient's and doctor's determinations and needs, which are significant to their relationship, resides in how their interaction has been conceptualised and classified to date in the literature.

The categorisation of the medical encounter has been reduced to an arid theory, paradoxically losing the humanistic components of both partners, which ultimately are at the centre of the doctor-patient relationship. Because this (medical) relationship implies both the doctor's and patient's involvement, I argue that, by not being aware of and accepting the doctor-patient rapport as a dyad, there will always be an asymmetry in their interaction, and there will always exist a "sufferer"—the patient in a "doctor-centred" medicine, and the doctor in the "patient-centred" medicine. The general argument that I present resides in the neglected needs, rights or personality traits of each one. Ultimately, the patient and the doctor form a unit that cannot be reduced to one.

A dyad concerns two people who relate to each other and are in an interdependent dynamic responding to one another's input as part of their interaction. Moreover, their communication is dyadic, because each must shift from speaker to listener for an effective exchange of information [11]. If we transpose this into the medical context, a dyad aims to reach the appropriate therapeutic strategy for the patient's best outcome [12]. Therefore, what has been ignored until now, on the one hand, is the patient's particularities as an individual in the so-called disease-centred or physician-centred medicine and, on the other hand, the doctor's humane traits in the "patient-centred," considered humanistic medicine. These aspects, alongside the communication within the doctor-patient relationship, are crucial for an effective rapport to take place in the medical encounter. Therefore, if we dismiss the fact that "a physician and a patient make up a social system" [13, p. 820], we adopt an oblivious attitude that may affect both the patient's outcome and the physician's mental health.

2.1.2 Doctor-Patient Dyad Within the Decision-Making Process

One of the best "markers" of evaluating the doctor-patient interaction is looking at how the decision-making process is taking place. A few critical aspects should be discussed when analysing Marcum's decision-making models—paternalistic and authoritarian as the biomedical model and empathetic, collaborative and humanistic as the bio-psycho-social model—one of which regards the person from the doctor-patient rapport who is designated as "the source for all the inputs and integrative processes" [1, p. 131]. According to Marcum, this source is the physician—I will refer to this part as the *power ratio dimension*. The second aspect is the association he makes between types of decision-making approaches (paternalistic vs. collaborative) and perspectives-taking from a reductionist point of view (considering the patient only as a biological organism, "disease-centred" medicine or evidence-based medicine) or humanistic (patient-centred medicine)—that may lead to a paradigm.

Firstly, a paternalistic approach can be made in a caring, humane manner considering a patient's values, and is therefore humanistic, as proven in Chap. 3 A Semantic Relationism Approach to Doctor-Patient Relationship. Secondly, a humanistic approach can interfere with a patient's values, needs or expectations about showing empathy (i.e. sensitive vs. pragmatic patients), and could be considered non-humanistic as it is doctor-centred instead of patient-centred, since the physician follows their own predefined model. They think they know what is best for the patient, not what that patient expects or needs to receive. This claim would most probably not be understood by Western country doctors, but it does have significant relevance, in Eastern European countries, mainly post-communist like Romania [14], Croatia [15] or low- to medium-developed countries [16]. These differences reside in cultural and past political contexts where social hierarchy dictates interpersonal rapport with educated people, like doctors or lawyers were more knowledgeable and more respected and trusted when it came to their input on professional-specific problems. However, when these countries were liberated from authoritarian and dictatorship regimes, society, and especially the younger population, has suffered a significant shift. Due to the increasing number of highly educated people in current times, these hierarchical considerations no longer define how human reports are made. Adding to this social inheritance and patients' easy access to information through the internet, doctors are less capable of establishing a collaborative approach using the obsolete paternalistic paradigm than Western physicians.

2.1.2.1 The Power Ratio Dimension

Marcum's decision-making models are based on the power ratio between the doctor and the patient. Accordingly, there can be a rapport between powerful and powerless agents or between empowering and empowered agents. In the powerful-powerless relationship, the physician is the active agent who makes clinical decisions, whereas the patient is passive and complies with whatever the doctor decides (traditional paternalistic model): "the physician is the source for all the inputs and integrative processes" [1, p. 131] or the patient is part of the clinical decision process in the sense of covering the informed consent aspect that needs to be fulfilled. In both situations, the patient is passive and the physician is the decision maker. In contrast, in the empowering-empowered rapport, the physician communicates the options and possible outcomes for each, whereas the patient is the decision maker—"it involves the expert knowledge of both the patient and physician" (ibid.).

According to Marcum, the decision-making approach from the powerful-powerless model is inevitably paternalistic and, as a consequence, part of the biomedical model of practice. In the second case, the empowering-empowered model offers the patient the chance to include their subjective perspective, and as such, it determines a collaborative aspect of the doctor-patient relationship. For Marcum, this rapport falls implicitly under the bio-psycho-social model of practicing medicine [1].

The paternalistic approach is often considered the worst, and the collaborative the most appreciated and encouraged [17, 18]. The central aspects of these categories are how the doctor relates to the patient and investigates the human body as a mechanical living organism (biomedical model) or as a mechanical living organism alongside its humane experiences, psychological and social (biopsychosocial model). Within the past few decades, many scholars have pleaded for the humanistic approach [1, 3, 15, 17, 19–25]. Notwithstanding, neither perspective brings a balanced view, since all are based on a "one size fits all" principle. They do not address the root problem for a genuine doctor-patient interaction, which focusses on a transparent and positive rapport for both the doctor and the patient. Led by this principle, a doctor guides their behaviour towards a patient according to their own beliefs and applies them generically, hence *not* on what a particular patient would best respond to. The healthcare practitioners should adopt their approach according to the patient's set of beliefs and needs and not according to the doctor's frame of reference; be it "humanistic" or not.

2.1.3 The Quality-of-Care Crisis

> In response to the quality-of-care crisis, many physicians and healthcare professionals call for humanising the biomedical model upon which modern medical knowledge and practice are based. The result is a variety of humane or humanistic models from the biopsychosocial model to the narrative model, in which the patient's human dimension is reinstated into the patient-physician relationship. [1, p. v]

I consider Marcum's position incomplete, because doctors' logic and determination to adhere to a specific conceptual framework may reside in their medical training or their mentor's blueprint, closely dependent on their education [26–29]. Moreover, there are differences between younger patients and younger doctors, although they come from the same cultural and societal context. As mentors, doctors pass on old customs they have learned to younger generations. In other words, younger doctors came across a set of doctor-patient relationship habits or styles from senior doctors [30]. In contrast, younger patients in general do not embrace paternalistic attitudes or any of this kind of medical stance. In contrast, an older patient used to a paternalistic approach may see a doctor's humanistic approach as too soft, which may affect their medical relationship.

Either way, if their set of beliefs contrasts, a young doctor may choose a mentor's approach instead of the spirit they have trained in. Therefore, we can either speak about a vicious circle that leads the medical student to perpetuate the flaws of a detached approach or a virtuous circle that may be enhanced by future doctors concerned with more quality-of-care practice under the right precepts.

A doctor ought to overcome the need to classify his rapport with patients into rigid categories, which implies understanding the referential system of each patient. After all, this is what humane centeredness is, namely, not treating every person in the same manner but by observing the person in front of them and acknowledging their values and beliefs before engaging in any interaction.

Why should a doctor be interested in this aspect? Because they need to set the proper social context with the patient, which will foster qualitative communication in a medical system under time pressure. What is qualitative communication in the doctor-patient interaction? An exchange of medical information and knowledge that needs to be revealed from both sides, moderated by the doctor, for the patient's benefit, following the "help me to help you" principle. For this to happen, it is not sufficient to merely express this principle for a suitable informational exchange but rather a flexible attitude towards any patient.

Why is this important? Firstly, by adopting one of the doctor-patient interaction models based on the "one size fits all" principle, that doctor will not have a suitable approach to a patient's specific language. Therefore, that person will try to find an answer by randomly picking one option from various presented on non-medical social groups, be they online or offline in the medical waiting room, and completely dismiss conventional treatment provided by a specialist. We can consider this as a medical dropout with dramatic consequences, for example oncological patients choosing to be treated with natural remedies instead of standard treatment, because they were not satisfied with their relationship with the doctor [31–33]. Secondly, it will determine an obsolete doctor-centred medicine, which should not be confounded with a paternalistic approach.

I, therefore, claim that the quality-of-care crisis is caused by paternalism, understood as an authoritarian figure due to a lack of compassionate care in their relationship with the patient regardless of the paradigm they choose to understand the human body. To strengthen this claim, consider a paternalistic physician who can adopt a humanistic, compassionate approach, although they do not see the patient's biological pathology in conjunction with their psycho-social valences. Also, they may not consider that the patient's outcome is linked to the quality of their interaction and the humane support offered during hospitalisation. Despite this view, however, this physician remains faithful to the art of medicine.

2.1.4 *The Limit* of *and the Price* for *a Humanistic Model*

The humanistic medical model—with the valence of caring for a patient's affective aspect—should not be practiced as a golden rule. First, physicians do not share a common feature such as emotional openness or availability that could make them natural people-person practitioners without emotionally fatiguing. Therefore, we cannot expect that emotional availability should be mandatory in the same way that clinical reasoning or judgement is. Second, clinical practice is time-consuming on its own without mentioning the time and effort, a sensitive situation could mean for a rigorous and "healthy" clinical judgement. Finally, the doctor is the clinical practitioner and part of the healthcare system.

The desire to become a medical practitioner, in general, could be determined by the curiosity of discovering the wonders of the human body and not the complexity of the human mind and its implications on the body—if we think of the psychoneuroimmunological branch of medicine or the placebo effect (in-depth examined in Chap. 7). Conversely, those who practice psychiatry may embrace the hard explanations of the mind (the genetics and the physiology of the brain with its neurohormones that explain certain behaviours) or focus more on the phenomenological experience of the patient and the environmental determinations that can explain their deviations, that is post-traumatic stress disorder that may lead to pathology. As such, the humane and humanistic elements that ought to be part of the medical act should be seen from the perspective of compassionate care and open communication skills that can facilitate an effective exchange of information between the patient and the physician: the "help me to help you" approach. For this to happen, an open qualitative dialogue is needed, and the person responsible for creating this setting is the healthcare giver. Being empathetic may be a fatiguing internal action, whilst being compassionate requires a personal endeavour that some may never be capable of without stumbling in the process of controlled detachment from their own experiences. The line is fine.

2.1.4.1 Can the Entire Medical System Be Humanistic?

Juliette Ferry-Danini's [34] view on humanism in clinical practice is based on expanding the general understanding of medicine by combining the health system and all its actors and medicine as both an art and science; in this way, she excludes individuality from being a pivotal factor that may lead to humanistic medicine. She does not defend a position against biomedicine but incorporates the individual's place in "the health system and its multiple devices (administrative, legal, financial, etc.)" as having the power "to produce good health outcomes" [34, p. 74]. She focusses on the medical system in which the encounter occurs rather than the doctor-patient relationship, and thus her marker for humanistic medicine regards the "outcomes-oriented approach" [34, p. 73], which falls under the system's responsibility and not on the individuals. I counterargue this position, since the system comprises individuals and the relations they form through a natural skillset, and focussing on administrative, legal and financial changes to design a humanistic medicine is to regiment inter-transferable skills.

Specialised medical literature has often been taught to equate paternalism with authority and humanism with empathy as if these are absolute truths. However, if we look at the above arguments, which show that these connections do not hold, it proves that they are not universal laws but assumptions that can vary depending on the context. Therefore, the association between paternalism and authority, and humanism and empathy that a priori could be labelled as axioms are, de facto, widely held assumptions. This shift from generalisation to context-specific correlations invites further exploration of the conditions under which these patterns hold true or deviate.

2.2 Cognitive Knowledge Gaps in Medical Care

Within the philosophy of medicine literature, significant emphasis has been put on concepts such as health and disease, suffering and illness, decision making. One concept that has been disregarded is the mental processing dimension from the patient and the physician perspectives because of the web of thoughts built on the patient's and physician's knowledge, expectations, beliefs and spiritual determinations. Consequently, the dynamics between the two have not been analysed in-depth, except for "the neuroscience behind the doctor-patient relationship" by studying it at the level of the placebo effect [35]. It is instrumental in analysing this web of mental processing dimensions on both sides (physician's and patient's) to better acknowledge its role at a more profound level and understand its importance. I claim that the physician's and the patient's mental processes are self-standing; they interplay and depend on each other. This cognitive interaction transposed in behaviour and dialogue has considerable impact both on the patient's outcome and the physician's mental health. From the physician's mental processing perspective, the clinical decision-making process has been thoroughly addressed, whereas metalevel thinking has only been discussed within the framework of storing and retrieving information through metacognitive skills. The question that emerges from this stance is: What has been left out in this "cognitive processing" dimension, and why is it essential to find out?

A distinction between cognitive layers of thinking in intelligent agents must be stated from the beginning. There are three pillars of cognition manifesting on separate levels. They are self-standing and continuously interplaying. These are the (1) ground-level, (2) the object-level and (3) meta-level thinking [36]. An intelligent agent chooses what actions to take based on the ability to reach their objectives. Ground-level cognition refers to basic mental processes involved in perception or attention, whilst object-level cognition entails memory or decision-making tasks [37]. Each level of cognition serves as a building block for higher-order cognitive functions where the actions that occur at the ground level determine a cyclical pattern that influences the object-level. On a metalevel, thinking involves monitoring and controlling computational activities at the higher level and it implies reflecting on and controlling one's own reasoning. Through the cognitive control feature, metalevel thinking enhances the quality of decision making by allocating effort towards determining the extent of reasoning required rather than just focussing on the actions to be taken. It is a cognitive tool that measures the balance between computational actions (object-level) and behavioural actions (ground-level).

Therefore, these levels involve one's perceptions and, respectively, one's action towards achieving specific goals based on the perceived inputs. An input (perception) and output (action) continuous loop determines a decision-making process. The metalevel defines the process of thinking about this specific loop, metareasoning, or metacognitive processing. The sequence is an ongoing and changing course of action where each process, thinking and metathinking, and their subsequent parts overlap. Metareasoning relies on the essential elements of reasoning, whilst reasoning is based on the ground and object levels of cognition [38].

Even though there are well-established categories of doctor-patient interaction following paternalistic, transactional or shared decision making, there is a gap in understanding the particularities that patients may present. Imagine that we label patients according to the above-mentioned types of doctor-patient relationships, however, if we do so, we miss the full picture of the patient's capacity to engage in unaware metacognitive processing (thinking about one's own thinking) concerning their own mental take on their medical condition.[1]

Let us consider the patient who projects themselves on someone else's situation, someone with a disease that "looks like" theirs, without filtering the information concerning their condition. This patient will be oblivious to possible solutions they may try to treat or deal with their condition. For example suppose the patient reads on the internet that someone with the same diagnosis died. In that case, they will not

[1] Systematically examined in Chaps. 3 A Semantic Relationism Approach to Doctor-Patient Relationship., 6 Extended Mind Theory and the Doctor-Patient Relationship, 7 Placebo: Evidence of the Patient's Extended Mind, 8 Metacognition from A to Z And Its Relevance in Medicine and 9 Metacognitive Implications on Physiological Disorders.

try to use the remaining chances that might prevent them from this scenario if they are not metacognitively processing their mental attitude linked to that condition. On the other hand, some patients filter all they gather and then decide what is best for them with the clinical practitioner.

First and foremost, it is essential to comprehend that the psychological burden on the patient who has just received bad news may be related to their beliefs about that diagnosis and not to what that diagnosis actually means for a doctor in medical terms. An ulcer might affect one patient minimally, whilst another might be significantly affected by it, possibly due to their past experiences with someone who had the same diagnosis. Therefore, if the physician sticks to the biomedical, mechanistic approach, they may be oblivious to the variety of psychological reactions displayed by the patient, which in turn may be detrimental to the patient-doctor dialogue. Consequently, the physician will neglect the image that the patient projects of their disease.

2.2.1 Metacognition and Self-Reflection in Medicine

Humans experience the first signs of metacognitive processing during the first years of life through the mental development stage [39]. The most noticeable metacognitive actions are planning, monitoring and reviewing mental actions to achieve an objective. A child does all these automatically due to a new logical setup, whereas adults can use metacognition explicitly as a tool to achieve a specific goal.

Since patients frequently respond emotionally to their medical conditions, it is important to address the necessity for therapeutic dialogue that assists them in understanding their own mental reactions and actions [9, 40]. Although there are a large number of studies concerned with patients' emotions, the literature has overlooked the cognitive and metacognitive dimension of the doctor-patient relationship, with notable exceptions found primarily in the field of psychiatry, especially concerning the treatment of schizophrenic patients [41]—a narrow and specialised view despite the relevance that metacognitive processes may exhibit across all medical disciplines. To understand emotions means to understand one's own thinking (metacognition). Therefore, adhering to developing the inherent tool of the metacognitive process instead of a generic, one-size-fits-all approach could transform the doctor-patient relationship into a conduit for effective communication with possible improved health outcomes. This redirected focus from the outside world to the inner cognitive world of the patient through metacognitive strategies requires doctors to foster a metacognitive mindset, not only by encouraging patients to reflect on their mental states but also by engaging in self-reflection regarding their own decision-making processes and interactions with patients. In this respect, conscious effort is essential (as outlined in Chaps. 8, 9 and 10); without a deliberate approach, the metacognitive process would be incomplete in the sense that "not setting a clear goal" would impede a fully aware process in managing the patient's optimal care.

In short, within the doctor-patient relationship, the working definition for "metacognition" used throughout the thesis is "thinking about one's thinking" has developed on two layers; one is the physicians', and the other one is the patient's cognitive processes. Each one relates to self-thinking but follows different goals: the patient's best health outcome and the physician's mental health. The distinction lies in the strategies each party engages with in order to achieve this goal, since their roles are defined by their power level (the physician assumes the empowering role, whilst the patient is empowered).

Therefore, from the physician's standpoint, I consider that metacognition is the cognitive process of monitoring and controlling their own cognition with an effect on their relationship with the patient and, implicitly, with an impact on the patient's positive health outcome as well as on their cognitive and personal implication in the process. Regarding the patient, metacognition is the patient's cognitive process of monitoring and controlling their own cognition, which affects their positive health outcome, influenced by the physician's approach. Hence, they both influence the medical rapport; the only difference is that the medical professional should be the one who is aware of the process and, thus, of the role they have in further developing the patient's metacognitive abilities for the benefit of their medical evolution. In achieving this, the physician should monitor and control their own mental activities within their relationship with the patient.

To return to the main argument, the shift in mentalities, given by the introduction of metacognition in medicine, may facilitate the switch from a biomedical-guided or biopsychosocial-guided approach to a relationship-centred medical practice. Experienced medical practitioners are professional experts, who customise and tailor statistical evidence to ascertain whether it fits the bedside data or not, and in doing so, they often mix evidence with expertise through intuitive judgments. Experts are poised to reflect on the reliability of their intuitions, especially when these occasionally misfire. Although intuition is, in fact, a telling instance of metacognition, its relevance has been explored only in the decision-making process that implies the diagnosis and not within the cognitive interaction with patients. Moreover, there is scarce information in the medical literature regarding metacognition in medical practice [41–44] or medical education [45–47] and none tackle metacognition in doctors interacting with patients or metacognition for the doctor's mental health or the patient's best health outcome. This fact prompts the question of how doctor-patient interactions are framed, from a cognitive perspective, within BMM-guided or BPSM-guided practices.

I claim that a biopsychosocial-guided practice can be metacognitive only inherently. The BPS-guided practitioner is mainly concerned with completing the entire picture of what constitutes the unicity of that specific individual, namely, the psyche and the social aspect, as well as the biological. Hence, the BPS-guided practitioner is inherently trying to find a way to mentally reach that specific patient using metacognitive skills to monitor, control and adapt their approach. By doing so, they focus on getting the answers they need to offer the best care for that specific patient, which may play a significant role in finding the proper treatment for their needs. Hence, the BPSM-guided practitioner's approach is being permanently adjusted due to the unicity of the patient in front of them. There are no guidelines for this kind of interaction, but the physician uses an internal compass to determine how to interact with the patient to gather all the pertinent information needed for the most appropriate treatment. Therefore, this stance proves that the BPS-guided doctor uses metacognitive processing as an inherent, automatic mental activity motivated by finding other traits that may have contributed to the occurrence of that specific medical condition: an approach that may impact the outcome of the patient. In contrast, a BMM-guided practitioner is not concerned about how to reach pertinent information other than the biological one.

2.3 Discussion

In looking at the doctor–patient relationship from a cognitive perspective, I aim to shed light on the limitations of current medical models—both the biomedical and biopsychosocial—for being too rigid and often falling short of genuinely centring the patient. In reflecting on the doctor-patient relationship through a cognitive lens, I aim to point out the shortcomings of dominant models in medical practice—namely, the biomedical and biopsychosocial approaches—which, despite their influence, often prove too rigid and fail to fully account for the individual needs and perspectives of patients.

The recognition of the cognitive and metacognitive processes underlying the doctor-patient relationship offers a deeper understanding of its dynamics and suggests that to really improve modern healthcare, it requires a shift in how medical professionals are trained to think about and engage with their patients.

Nonetheless, implementing such an approach raises several challenges with the most important being the development of the skills and mindset necessary for future doctors to adapt their approach to the patient, which is a different mentality from the one they found with their mentors; this, of course, means a type of medical education reform through systematic changes. Furthermore, the concern regarding the practicality of applying it in busy clinical settings, where time and resources are often limited, may be false, since once the skillsets are there, they become an automatic cognitive reflex.

2.4 Conclusion

This chapter argues for the rethinking of the doctor-patient relationship through a model that is more responsive to the patient's individual needs and the cognitive processes behind medical interactions. At the heart of this proposal is an emphasis on cognitive and metacognitive processes—those reflective mechanisms through which both doctors and patients interpret, evaluate and respond to the clinical encounter, thus moving beyond the formal structures of the biomedical and biopsychosocial models, which often fall short in practice, and instead cultivate a dynamic, context-sensitive relationship grounded in awareness.

Future research must engage with the practical dimensions of this challenge: identifying the skills required to support metacognitive sensitivity in clinical settings, examining how these skills shape patient care and professional judgment and assessing their broader impact on practitioner well-being. If the ambition is truly patient-centred care adding to the medical professional's well-being, then the intellectual and emotional labour of medicine must be revalued—not as peripheral, but as central to ethical and effective practice.

References

1. Marcum JA (2008) An introductory philosophy of medicine. Humanizing modern medicine. Springer, Dordrecht. https://doi.org/10.1007/978-1-4020-6797-6
2. Stewart M, Belle Brown J, Weston W, Mcwhinney IR, Mcwilliam CL, Freeman TR (2014) Patient-centered medicine: transforming the clinical method. Radcliffe Publishing, London
3. Genuis QIT (2021) A genealogy of autonomy: freedom, paternalism, and the future of the doctor–patient relationship. J Med Philos 46:330–349
4. Engel GL (1997) From biomedical to biopsychosocial: being scientific in the human domain. Psychosomatics 38:521–528
5. Engel GL (1977) The need for a new medical model: a challenge for biomedicine. Science 196:129–136
6. Pellegrino E (2005) The "telos" of medicine and the good of the patient. In: Clinical bioethics, pp 21–32
7. Pellegrino ED, Thomasma DC (1993) The virtues in medical practice. Oxford University Press, New York
8. Komrad MS (1983) A defence of medical paternalism: maximising patients' autonomy. J Med Ethics 9:38–44
9. Reach G (2014) Patient autonomy in chronic care: solving a paradox. Patient Prefer Adherence 8:15–24
10. Beauchamp T, Childress J (2019) Principles of biomedical ethics, 8th edn. Oxford University Press, New York
11. Brauer K, Proyer RT (2019) Dyadic effects. In: Encyclopedia of personality and individual differences. Springer, Cham, pp 1–5
12. Halpern J (2001) From detached concern to empathy. Humanizing medical practice. Oxford University Press, New York
13. Henderson LJ (1935) Physician and patient as a social system. N Engl J Med 212:819–823
14. Florea GP (2019) Philosophy of medicine in post-communist Romania. From a paternalistic model toward a patient-centered medicine. In: Florea GP, Cernica V (eds) Reality and appearance, evidence and probability. University of Bucharest Publishing House, Bucharest, pp 55–72
15. Murgic L, Hébert PC, Sovic S, Pavlekovic G (2015) Paternalism and autonomy: views of patients and providers in a transitional (post-communist) country. BMC Med Ethics. https://doi.org/10.1186/S12910-015-0059-Z
16. Málaga G, Romero ZO, Málaga AS, Cuba-Fuentes S (2017) Shared decision making and the promise of a respectful and equitable healthcare system in Peru. Z Evid Fortbild Qual Gesundhwes 123–124:81–84

17. Des Ordons ALR, De Groot JM, Rosenal T, Viceer N, Nixon L (2018) How clinicians integrate humanism in their clinical workplace—'Just trying to put myself in their human being shoes'. Perspect Med Educ 7:318–324
18. Hagen KB (2020) Lessons on causality from clinical encounters with severely obese patients. In: Rethinking causality, complexity and evidence for the unique patient: a causehealth resource for healthcare professionals and the clinical encounter. Springer, Cham, pp 149–165
19. Baltonado J, Cymet T (2017) Can the humanities humanize health care? J Am Osteopath Assoc 117:273–275
20. Card AJ (2022) The biopsychosociotechnical model: a systems-based framework for human-centered health improvement. Health Syst 12(4):387–407
21. Bleakley A (2020) Routledge handbook of medical humanities. Routledge, Abingdon
22. Thibault GE (2019) Humanism in medicine: what does it mean and why is it more important than ever? Acad Med 94:1074–1077
23. Schramme T (2015) New perspectives on paternalism and health care. Springer, Cham. https://doi.org/10.1007/978-3-319-17960-5
24. Marcum JA (2008) Reflections on humanizing biomedicine. Perspect Biol Med 51:392–405
25. Marcum JA (2021) P7 medicine: humanizing systems medicine. Teorema 40:215–231
26. Cuff PA, Vanselow N, Behavioral C, Sciences S, Neuroscience B, Health B (2004) Improving medical education. National Academies Press, Washington, DC. https://doi.org/10.17226/10956
27. Austin J, Bentkover J, Chait L (2016) Leading strategic change in an era of healthcare transformation. Springer, Cham. https://doi.org/10.1007/978-3-319-30776-3
28. Skorton D, Bear A (2018) The integration of the humanities and arts with Sciences, engineering, and medicine in higher education. The National Academies Press, Washington, DC. https://doi.org/10.17226/24988
29. Shaham D, Kandel L, Gural A (2011) Establishing a medical humanities program in Israel: challenges and solutions. Eur Leg 16:307–315
30. Răduca I (2020) Doctors' biases and common laws may lead to errors. Dissertation, University of Bucharest
31. Shumay DM, Maskarinec G, Kakai H, Gotay CC (2001) Why some cancer patients choose complementary and alternative medicine instead of conventional treatment. J Fam Pract 12:1067
32. Frenkel M, Ben-Arye E, Cohen L (2010) Communication in cancer care: discussing complementary and alternative medicine. Integr Cancer Ther 9:177–185
33. Adams M, Jewell AP (2007) The use of complementary and alternative medicine by cancer patients. Int Semin Surg Oncol 4:10
34. Ferry-Danini J (2018) A new path for humanistic medicine. Theor Med Bioeth 39:57–77
35. Benedetti F (2010) Feeling sick: a combination of bottom-up and top-down events. In: The patient's brain. Oxford University Press, Oxford, pp 53–100
36. Nelson TO, Narens L (1990) Metamemory: a theoretical framework and new findings. Psychol Learn Motiv 26:125–173
37. Ackerman R, Thompson VA (2017) Meta-reasoning: monitoring and control of thinking and reasoning. Trends Cogn Sci 21:607–617
38. Cox MT, Raja A (eds) (2011) Metareasoning: thinking about thinking. The MIT Press, Cambridge, MA
39. Flavell JH (1979) Metacognition and cognitive monitoring. A new area of cognitive-developmental inquiry. Am Psychol 34:906–911
40. Gürhan N, Beşer NG, Polat Ü, Koç M (2019) Suicide risk and depression in individuals with chronic illness. Community Ment Health J 55:840–848
41. Dimaggio G, Semerari A, Carcione A, Nicolo G, Procacci M (2007) Psychotherapy of personality disorders: metacognition, states of mind and interpersonal cycles. Routledge, London
42. Coulacoglou C, Saklofske DH (2017) Metacognition, empathy, and cognitive biases in schizophrenia and OCD. In: Psychometrics and psychological assessment. Elsevier, Amsterdam, pp 131–153

43. Hertzog C (2002) Metacognition in older adults: implications for application. In: Perfect TJ, Schwartz BL (eds) Applied metacognition. Cambridge University Press, pp 169–196
44. Marcum JA (2012) An integrated model of clinical reasoning: dual-process theory of cognition and metacognition. J Eval Clin Pract 18:954–961
45. Mark Q (2006) Intuition and metacognition in medical education: keys to developing expertise, Springer series on medical education. Springer, New York. https://doi.org/10.4103/1357-6283.143784
46. Kosior K, Wall T, Ferrero S (2019) The role of metacognition in teaching clinical reasoning: theory to practice. Educ Health Prof 2:108
47. Nazarieh M (2016) A brief history of metacognition and principles of metacognitive instruction in learning. Best J Humanit Arts Med Sci 2:61–64

Chapter 3
A Semantic Relationism Approach to Doctor-Patient Relationship

3.1 Introduction

In the field of philosophy of medicine, the words "model," "paradigm" or "approach" are frequently used and often interchangeable [1, p. 448]. They are employed in conjunction with concepts like "biomedical," biopsychosocial" or "humanistic" and linked with specific epistemological (objective or subjective knowledge), metaphysical (mechanistic monism, or dualism/holism) or ethical (empathic detached concern, empathic care) considerations [2, p. 11].

I detach from this interchangeable usage for they need a better conceptualisation and, consequently, consistency in grasping a medical act based on the following two aspects: (1) a doctor can have a biomedical understanding of the patient whilst their approach towards the patient can be a humanistic one in terms of ethical considerations, thus manifesting empathy or compassion in the relationship with that patient and (2) a humanistic physician can adopt a shared-decision approach with either an empathetic detached concern or empathetic care. I endorse both claims through the intrinsic values the physician may embrace, which are or are not dependent on external factors. A rigid framework was built for these terms, models, paradigms or approaches. Consequently, the derived classification, humanistic, the BPSM, or non-humanistic, the BMM, becomes a reference point in rigidly labelling physicians according to a specific model that one would adopt. This conceptual rigidity creates confusion, since specific attributes shape a particular model, and none of them is to be assigned to the other, as I shall demonstrate below. Similarly, the same conceptual rigidity in classifying models of medical care may divide medical professionals into the same two categories: humanistic and non-humanistic.

Another essential aspect that should be discussed is that patients can adopt a specific "mental model" related to their medical condition (as discussed in Sect. 4.3. Models). In other words, patients may unknowingly follow the same models as medical professionals. More precisely, following this perspective, patients may not

G.-P. Florea, *Metacognition and Medical Humanities in Medical Education*, New Paradigms in Healthcare, https://doi.org/10.1007/978-3-032-01070-4_3

wish to address their psychological or sociological dimensions, because they may not consider them relevant even after they have been presented with these concepts. Therefore, they may agree upon a biomedical vision for treating their disease rather than a psychological and social add-on. Similarly, the same patients may not appreciate an empathic approach from their doctor, and they may also wish that the doctor exhibits paternalistic power and makes decisions on their behalf. Thus, if the so-called humanistic physicians have to build a good relationship with these patients, they would have to manifest empathic detached concern instead of empathic care; these patients would expect a straight answer to their medical condition rather than a complex dialogue on psychological and social layers related to their disease. A problem that derives from this is that, so far as the literature goes, a piece of evidence regarding patients' typologies is scarce. The research focus in this respect was mainly to show what models doctors should adopt [2] instead of observing what each patient might need according to their beliefs. Therefore, a starting point in constructing a model of practice should be understanding how patients think and how the physician should address each of the typologies, not based on a general understanding but contextually patient dependent.

This is the depth that proper patient-centred medicine (PCM) should reach. As generally accepted, the humanistic approach cannot be presented as a golden rule, since it would imply a prerequisite that physicians should manifest, depending on patients' needs, beliefs or intrinsic values. In addition, this approach would be better understood if we put both participants in the medical encounter in conjunction and do not take them separately. The humanistic approach centred on the patient is beneficial and desirable, but it must be contextualised to each patient, because some patients prefer a more pragmatic and emotionally detached approach. Therefore, an appropriate and relative endowment is needed for each case.

In doctor-patient interaction, the problem related to how the "relationship" may be defined comes across inevitably. To analyse the "relationship" concept in the medical encounter, we should consider it a binomial comprised of the doctor and the patient. This binomial can also be viewed as a semantic relation through Fine's [3] approach to semantic relationism. Therefore, the two constituents of the binomial, the doctor and the patient, can be seen as variables that range over the same domain (the medical environment). Conventionally, we can refer to the doctor as variable "*x*" and the patient as variable "*y*." The context in which we address the two variables is the medical encounter, since any analysis outside this context would not serve the primary purpose of the medical act.

The following discussion will be on the relationism between the two variables as part of the expression, "The doctor and the patient must have a good medical relationship for the patient's best health outcome." To analyse the words "doctor" and "patient" and their connection within the semantic relationism theory, we must first establish their meaning and roles. Therefore, the first section will examine what I call "the binominal implicit rejection" and the second "the binomial's erroneously applied humanity." The former covers the implicit definitions of doctor and patient within the biomedical medicine model. In contrast, the latter covers the meanings of doctor and patient, implicitly adopted by the biopsychosocial model. Through this analysis, I wish to show that none of the most used models in medicine are patient centred and that the concept of humanity is erroneously applied, since none of them is taking the patient's set of beliefs into account, but a general understanding of humane values. In other words, I claim that one model is not different from the other, because both focus on what set of beliefs physicians must adopt, and not that they should adapt their approach according to the patient's needs. Thus, I stress that both models (the biomedical and the humanistic) are ambiguous and falsely assumed and, consequently, that a new flexible model for the doctor-patient relationship should be provided on the true relationship-centred principle. This original approach should satisfy each binomial doctor-patient component's intrinsic and extrinsic features based on Kit Fine's theory concerning semantic relationism.

3.2 Semantic Relationism in the Doctor-Patient Relationship

Firstly, we should set the formal symbolism we refer to. As such, "x" will be the symbol assigned to the word "doctor," considered as one of the variables within the expression "$x \wedge y$," and the symbol "y" assigned to the word "patient" in the same construct "$x \wedge y$." Subsequently, following Fine's symbolism, clarification ought to be made, namely, why "x" and "y" are taken as variables instead of constants. Although "x" may have the same external meaning (a doctor is a doctor within any model in medicine), "x" from a particular model differs from "x" that adopts a different model of medical practice due to its ascribed *intrinsic* features. Conversely, although the word "patient" has the same general meaning, it changes depending on the inherent features or the set of beliefs the patient may have.

Secondly, the definitions of "x" and "y" must be clearly stated from the beginning. Objectively, I prefer establishing impartial definitions for each binomial component. This approach is underpinned by deliberately excluding any value-laden propositions derived from the prevailing models. Henceforth, I shall denote the ensuing definitions as neutral, devoid of any inherent biases derived from the guiding principles underpinning prevalent models, whether biomedical or humanistic. For "x" (the doctor), the formal neutral definition would be a licensed, active medical professional, specialised in a general or specific medical branch that conducts medical examinations, who makes diagnoses, prescribes, and gives treatments, substance based and/or interventional based (surgical or mechanical) and considers preventive care by applying methods and treatments for specific conditions. The definition assigning meaning to the variable "y" (representing the patient) posits that a patient is an individual afflicted with an illness and/or undergoing treatment for a particular ailment, injury or disorder.

Because neither of the most used models in medicine (biomedical and biopsychosocial) offer explicit definitions of the doctor or the patient, we should extract one for each based on the models' core concepts within the following two sections.

3.3 The Binomial Implicit Rejection Theory

In this section, I explain “the binomial implicit rejection theory” based on the inadequacies found in the biomedical model (BMM). Therefore, all aspects presented in this section will be related to the BMM alone.

According to Marcum [2], the practitioner of the biomedical model follows the subsequent laws:

> [T]he patient is reduced to a physical body composed of separate body parts that occupy a machine-world. The physician’s emotionally detached concern is to identify the patient’s diseased body part and to treat or replace it, using the latest scientific and technological advances in medical knowledge sanctioned by the medical community. The outcome of this intervention is to cure the patient, thereby saving the patient from permanent injury or possibly death (…) The physician’s concern for the patient is detached from the emotions of either the physician or patient. [2, pp. 10, 13]

Starting from this definition, I add to the neutral definition the missing pieces that result from Marcum’s description to provide the meaning of “doctor” and “patient” in the BMM model. Therefore, a doctor is a licensed, active medical professional specialised in a general or specific medical branch who conducts medical examinations, makes diagnoses, prescribes and gives treatments, substance-based and/or interventional-based (surgical or mechanical), and considers preventive care by applying methods and treatments for specific conditions whilst manifesting an emotionally detached concern, using the latest scientific and technological developments in medicine, endorsed by the medical community. Therefore, I will term this definition as denoting the “biomedical doctor.”

An observation that one can draw from this definition is that an addition to the humane aspect of the doctor was made, more precisely, a firm assertion on the lack of the humane aspect regarding the doctor’s net delineation from the patient through “an emotionally detached concern.” On the other hand, based on previous observations, the patient has no value given to the humane aspect.

Hence, if the neutral definition gave the external determinants of a doctor (acquired knowledge and practical skills), the definition based on the BMM’s description confers the general intrinsic features (examples) starting from the premise that all doctors who see the body as a mechanical living organism have the same extrinsic features based on the expression “an emotionally detached concern.” I argue against this point and bring further clarification built on the argument that any human interaction implies social interaction triggered by motor and emotional behaviour based on social stimuli through facial expressions, prosodic vocalisations and body language [4, 5]. To say that doctors who adopt a biomedical model, “biomedical (or non-humanistic) doctors,” are manifesting an “emotionally detached concern,” one would understand that these types of doctors would not manifest emotional care and be completely detached from another person’s direct or indirect emotional expression. Some humans would not have the mirror-neuron system if that were the case. However, evidence does not support this [6–8], except in instances where specific neurological and/or psychiatric pathologies exist [9]. One cannot assume that doctors generally suffer from any of those mentioned above, socially inflicting pathologies that block the social stimuli connected with emotions. The assumption that doctors who practice medicine adopting the biomedical model would manifest an "emotionally detached concern" is not adequate; hence, the definition of the doctor that follows from the description of the biomedical model is ungrounded and conjectural.

In defining the variable "*y*", the patient, within the biomedical approach, we must follow the same approach, starting from the neutral to the more specific meaning. As mentioned before, the neutral definition for the patient is an individual afflicted with an illness and/or undergoing treatment for a particular ailment, injury, or disorder. From the description of the biomedical model alone, one can understand that "the patient is reduced to a physical body composed of separate body parts that occupy a "machine-world" [2, p. 10]. Therefore, within the BMM approach, the patient would be an individual afflicted with an illness and/or undergoing treatment for a particular ailment, injury, or disorder whilst being reduced to a physical body of separate parts that occupy a "machine-world". Therefore, from this perspective, the variable "*y*" would range over the following properties: *a physically ill body reduced to its parts*. These properties have a quantitative value measured externally (medical knowledge, epistemologically based). Hence, properties attributed to "*y*" are extrinsic.

Concerning the word "relationship," Marcum considers that "the patient's relationship to a physician is passive. The physician is the authoritative figure with the knowledge and power to save the patient. Thus, the physician's relationship with a patient is one of dominance, as represented by paternalism" [2, p. 13]. Therefore, the conjunction between the doctor and the patient, $x \wedge y$, has the following properties: asymmetrical, where "*y*" is passive (the patient), and "*x*" is dominant, thus paternal.

Nevertheless, I claim that taken separately, be it outside the doctor-patient relationship or within the doctor-patient relationship, "*y*" could take different values. Therefore, a distinction between theoretical and context-dependent representations must be made. I call the "non-contextual patient" the theoretical representation, namely, a general understanding or meaning of the word "patient" as presented above. I also refer to the "contextual patient" as the alternatives patients can ascribe depending on their intrinsic features. In the case of a "non-contextual patient," "*y*" will take the same values as for any given "*y*," whereas, in a "contextual patient," the values that "*y*" will ascribe will be contingent on the intrinsic features that "*y*" could manifest. Hence, the non-contextual patient "*y*" will have the same extrinsic features as those presented in the BMM definition, and there will be no intrinsic value, since there is none that this definition offers. On the other hand, the contextual patient symbolised through "*y*`" will take different values based on specific intrinsic features.

3.4 Breuer-Sigmund Though Experiment

Let us consider the following thought experiment.

3.4.1 Case 1.1

Frederic, a male patient, presents himself to the emergency care unit for severe headaches. The appointed doctor, Dr. Breuer, conducts the medical examination, diagnoses migraine, prescribes opioid therapy and takes into consideration prevention care whilst manifesting an emotionally detached concern. Throughout the medical examination and even after Dr. Breuer's input, Frederic does not ask anything, nor does he object to the doctor's method of approaching him. Frederic is pleased with Dr. Breuer's approach and prescribed treatment, for he followed it precisely.

3.4.2 Case 1.2

Sigmund, a male patient, presents himself to the emergency care unit for severe headaches. The appointed doctor, Dr. Breuer, conducts the medical examination, diagnoses migraine, prescribes opioid therapy and offers advice on prevention whilst manifesting an emotionally detached concern. After Dr. Breuer's input, Sigmund asks many questions to understand his symptoms; he complains about the excruciating pain affecting the quality of his life and the side effects the recommended therapy may have. He objects to Dr. Breuer's method of approaching him without empathy, let alone compassion. Dr. Breuer says he cannot do anything more than that for him. Sigmund leaves the room unhappy, accusing that the pain he is experiencing has increased, and he is unwilling to follow Dr. Breuer's indications and the prescribed medicine.

3.4.3 Case 1.1 Versus Case 1.2

This thought experiment aims to identify the features of each actor involved and then take them in conjunction to understand their dynamics. It is the dynamic on which the patient's compliance with the treatment and level of satisfaction is based, and the patient's expression manifested, in the end, reflects the effect of the interaction with the doctor. If we examine individual (personal) attributes separately and then conjointly, we reach the attributes of the relation between the two. I will refer to their beliefs as internal features, how they respond to one another as extrinsic features and the nature of their relationship as a qualitative indicator of their interaction.

From a theoretical perspective, based on the BMM's definition, the doctor-patient rapport in case 1.1 (C1.1) was non-humanistic, because Dr. Breuer had a biomedical approach in his clinical practice (but so did Frederic). Judging from Frederic's response, he was pleased with his doctor's attitude—the patient did comply with the prescribed treatment. We may then assert that in C.1.1, the Frederic-Breuer relationship was synergic and constructive, following Frederic's best health outcome. On the other hand, in case 1.2 (C1.2), Dr. Breuer manifested a biomedical approach, whilst Sigmund, the patient, was expecting a different one from all epistemological (subjective knowledge instead of objective knowledge), metaphysical (holistic rather than mechanical monism) and ethical (empathic care rather than an emotionally detached concern) levels. Sigmund had a biopsychosocial understanding of his medical condition—he asked questions to understand his symptoms; he complained about the excruciating pain that affected his life's quality and the possible side effects of Dr. Breuer's recommended therapy. Also, Sigmund was expecting at least an empathic attitude from his physician. He even objected to Dr. Breuer's attitude without receiving a change of attitude in return.

Most importantly, Sigmund left the room, stating a pain increase, and refused to follow the prescribed treatment. The bottom line is that Dr. Breuer failed to gain his patient's trust, because he did not address Sigmund's concerns. Theoretically, judging from the established definition, in C1.2, the doctor-patient rapport was asymmetrical and non-humanistic, and so was in reality. In conclusion, in C1.2, the Breuer-Sigmund relationship was antagonist and non-constructive, without following Sigmund's best health outcome based on his needs and expectations. Conversely, in C1.1, the Breuer-Frederic relationship was synergic and constructive, following Frederic's best health outcome, although the physician had a BMM-oriented approach.

Hence, what is common in both cases presented above is that the physician was practicing medicine based on BMM precepts. He reduced the patient to his medical condition, the migraine, and prescribed opioid therapy whilst manifesting an emotionally detached concern. The difference between the two presented situations is that the patient manifested a distinct understanding of his disease—in the first case, a BMM one, and a biopsychosocial model (BPSM) in the second. In short, C1.1 can be reduced to a BMM-BMM relationship, where the physician and the patient follow the same BMM approach, and C1.2 to BMM-BPSM, since the physician followed a BMM approach whilst the patient followed the BPSM. Correlating these observations with the patient's level of satisfaction and compliance with treatment in both cases, we can assert that for Frederic in C1.1, the physician had an appropriate approach, whilst in C1.2, that same approach was not appreciated by Sigmund, the different patient. Thus, it was not the physician who required a particular type of interaction with the patient but the patient himself. From this, it does not follow that the physician had the ideal approach. Still, it reveals that the dynamic of the doctor-patient relationship is based on the patients' vision regarding their condition, their needs and their expressed concerns. On a different level of understanding, one can observe that the physician expressed his set of beliefs openly without taking into account the patient's needs.

The first case had a positive outcome, whilst the second did not because the doctor did not seek to understand the patient's set of beliefs first and adapt his approach accordingly. To endorse these accounts, I will analyse the presented cases along Fine's (2007) semantic relationism lines. I will assign Dr. Breuer, the symbol "*b*", to Frederic, the patient from C1.1, the symbol "*f*" and Sigmund, the patient from C1.2, the symbol "*s*." The doctor-patient relationship from each of the two cases will be addressed using the conjunctive symbol "∧"; hence, the rapport between the variables will be represented through the expression "$b \wedge f$" and "$b \wedge s$," respectively. Also, by intrinsic feature, I refer to any non-relational characteristics that a variable may ascribe, directly or indirectly, and by extrinsic feature, I will refer to any trait a variable can assign within the binomial relation.

Starting from Marcum's interpretations, which are theoretical and non-contextual based, the relationship between the two variables "*b*" and "*f*" in C1.1 would carry a negative moral value, since the two are in an "asymmetrical rapport", $b \wedge f < 0$. Along this line, because "*b*" has a BMM approach, it implicitly follows that he manifests a paternal power over the patient; if we, in this context, assign to the word "power" a numerical value, it would be less than zero, because it carries a negative moral value when linked to BPSM and not to BMM, since the patient cannot manifest autonomy—thus, $b < 0$. On the other hand, "*f*" carries the extrinsic feature of being "passive," which, still under Marcum's BMM laws and in contrast with those associated with BPSM principles, can only assign a value less than or equal to 0; thus, $f \leq 0$: this derives from the same effect that the doctor's attitude, paternalistic, prevents patient's autonomy from being manifested. Marcum's observations will then be represented as $b \wedge f < 0$, where $b < 0, f \leq 0$, and $b \neq f$. Therefore, the expression carries an intrinsic negative feature due to the BMM's negative connotation assigned to the attribute of "asymmetrical relationship."

A significant question that must be asked at this point is as follows: If $b \wedge f < 0$, where $b < 0, f \leq 0, b \neq f$, thus a negative moral value, then why Frederic, from C1.1, was "pleased with Dr. Breuer's approach and prescribed treatment and followed it precisely"? It reflects a contradiction between theory, non-contextual, and context (C1.1). The answer stems from the presumptions one assumes when evaluating a theoretical model, not the intrinsic and extrinsic values that variables may ascribe contextually. Because Dr. Breuer was following a medical model considered non-humanistic (therefore with negative attributes), the conclusion that automatically follows is that the outcome is also negative, which is not the case in C1.1. This results from rejecting the existence of intrinsic features of "*f*" (the symbol assigned to Frederic, the patient from Case 1.1), an implicit understanding of the BMM's precepts. Consequently, it derives a falsely negative attribute assigned to the doctor-patient relationship based on the BMM's implicit principles. Contrary to this worldwide accepted understanding, C1.1 proves that BMM is not to be rejected in the proper context, provided by the patients' set of beliefs, thus their intrinsic features.

Therefore, if we analyse C1.1 from the patient's best interest and the level of satisfaction with the doctor's approach, C1.1 will take a different form, which is patient related. As such, the values assigned to the variables "*b*" and "*f*" must start from the end, namely, from the qualitative attributes that the "*f*" manifested externally (Frederic was pleased with Dr. Breuer's approach, and he complied with the prescribed treatment) and internally (Frederic himself shared the same vision as Dr. Breuer, BMM oriented). Therefore, due to the external features, the doctor-patient relationship will ascribe a positive value, $b \wedge f > 0$, where b and f, taken separately, can only have positive values. Moreover, by comparing the intrinsic features of both variables, namely, their sets of beliefs, they are on par—since both Breuer and Frederic adopt the same mechanical understanding of the migraines—then b will have the same intrinsic value as f, $b = f$. Therefore, the logical sequence will be $b \wedge f > 0$, where $b > 0, f > 0$, and $b = f$; thus, the result is also positive, as proven by Frederic's satisfaction related to Dr. Breuer's approach to him and treating his medical condition. In contrast, as derived from Marcum's perspective, we proved that b and f are asymmetrical. Thus, $b \wedge f < 0$, where $b < 0, f \leq 0$, and $b \neq f$. The contradiction signalled previously is therefore based on how the rapport is assessed from a theoretical understanding rather than a contextual one. Moreover, also because, implicitly, the patient's intrinsic features are not assessed, but only the extrinsic ones ("passive"), the indirect assumption that f cannot ascribe an intrinsic feature is inherent; derived from this is also the fact that f cannot ascribe the same feature as b does, since f does not have any internal features ascribed. Consequently, the external features that BMM implicitly assigns, non-contextually, "power" to b and "passivity" to f determine a negative value to $b \wedge f$, whereas, contextually, the exact conjunction may have a positive value.

Regarding C1.2, if we apply Marcum's laws, the expression will take the same negative value as in C1.1, because variable b has a BMM approach, $b \wedge s < 0$, where we only consider doctors' values, $b < 0$. The patient's value, s, cannot be assumed based on Marcum's assumption of the asymmetrical attribute of the relationship with Dr. Breuer, because Sigmund, compared to Frederic, is active, not passive. Therefore, going further with Marcum's rationale, s would ascribe a value greater than zero, $s > 0$. As such, the expression would be $b \wedge s < 0$, where $b < 0$, $s > 0$, and $b = s$ (based on the relational feature of power—extrinsic). Therefore, we reach a contradiction, because if $b < 0$ and $s > 0$, b cannot be equal to s. If we analyse based on intrinsic-extrinsic values, we understand that the patient's intrinsic values, in C1.2, differ from the physician's, because he has a BPSM understanding of their disease. Sigmund asks many questions to understand his symptoms; he complains about the excruciating pain affecting the quality of his life and the side effects the recommended therapy may have.

Therefore, from Fine's semantic relationism (not from Marcum's understanding), it implicitly follows that the intrinsic features of s are different from those of b, which means that $b \neq s$: the patient's satisfaction level and the qualitative indicator of the Dr. Breuer-Sigmund interaction, relational and thus external (such as "unhappy" and not complying with the prescribed treatment), confirms the doctor-patient interaction's negative result. In contradistinction, this was not the case with C1.1, where the overall result was positive on the same doctor BMM-based approach. Regarding the moral dimension, which is acknowledged given what the patient was expecting from his doctor, "He objects to Dr. Breuer's method of approaching him without empathy, let alone compassion", reflects the non-humanistic approach, in contrast with C1.1, where Frederic was not expecting otherwise than he received from Dr. Breuer. In conclusion, in C1.2, from the *true* patient-centred and relationship-centred perspectives, $b \wedge s$ will be negative but based on the patient's satisfaction level and compliance with the treatment. This negative value is reinforced by the doctor's inadaptation to the patient's needs and his set of beliefs; in other words, the added negative value reflects the physician's set of beliefs imposed on the interaction with the patient, because he cannot adapt to the patient's request to give him a humanistic perspective on all levels (epistemological, metaphysical and ethical) regarding his migraines, "Dr. Breuer tells him that he cannot do anything more than that for him." Therefore, even from a patient-centred view, $b \wedge s < 0$, where $b < 0$, $s > 0$, and $b \neq s$ with the variation that b is different from s, because s intrinsic features are different from those of b (b's intrinsic features, or set of beliefs, are BMM based, whilst f's intrinsic features are BPSM based).

In Marcum's attempt to advocate for humanistic medicine, the patient's intrinsic values are not considered, but only the external (passive/active) ones—see Table 3.1. A schematic representation of the values that the doctor and the patient can ascribe. Also, only the physician's nonrelational, intrinsic features are discussed and acknowledged. These observations reflect that the patient-doctor binomial is implicitly rejected within a rigid conceptual frame. The frame is inflexible, because it focusses on what a doctor should think instead of how a doctor should observe a patient to adapt their professional behaviour according to the patient's set of beliefs (internal features). Therefore, the doctor's own set of beliefs is implicitly accepted. At the same time, it proves that the doctor's behaviour should match the patient's needs and expectations when taken together—a conflict between their internal features manifested externally is then extinguished.

Table 3.1 A schematic representation of the values that the doctor and the patient can ascribe individually or taken together as are in the relationship, based on Kit Fine's Semantic Relationism applied in the medical context – both theoretical and contextual, where b is the doctor (Dr. Breuer), while f and s are the patients, Frederic and Sigmund, respectively, from each of the presented cases, C1.1 and C1.2

Case	Perspective	Ascribed values	Core principles		Ascribed values	Perspective	Case
1.1	Marcum's *BMM vs. BPSM*	$b \wedge f < 0$	Based on b **intrinsic** features (non-relational) *BMM approach*		$b \wedge s < 0$	Marcum's *BMM vs. BPSM*	1.2
		$b < 0$	Based on b **extrinsic** features (relational) *"power"*		$b < 0$		
		$f \leq 0$	Based on f/s **extrinsic** features (relational)		$s > 0$		
			"passive"	*"active"*			
		$b \neq f$	Based on b **and** f/s **extrinsic** features (relational)		$s = s$		
			power≠passive	***power=power***			
	Observation	-	-	If $b<0$, and $s>0$ then $b \neq s$ => Contradiction		Observation	
	Patient-centred	$b \wedge f > 0$	Based on b **and** f **extrinsic** features (relational) *Doctor-patient relationship*		$b \wedge s < 0$	Patient-centred	
		$b > 0$	Based on b **extrinsic** features (relational) *Doctor's attitude in rapport with the patient*		$b < 0$		
		$f > 0$	Based on f/s **extrinsic** features (relational)		$s > 0$		
		$b = f$	based on ***b*** **and** ***f/s*** **intrinsic** features (non-relational)		$b \neq s$		
			BMM=BMM	*BMM≠BPSM*			
	Observation	-	-	-	-	Observation	

3.5 Discussion: The Binomial's Humanity Erroneously Applied

In this section, I will explain why the binomial's humanity is erroneously applied based on the inadequacies found in the biopsychosocial model (BPSM). Therefore, all aspects presented in this section will be related to the biopsychosocial model alone.

When it comes to BPSM, we must first understand the bigger picture. Firstly, it belongs to the general group of humanistic medicine, amongst other variations, that is narrative medicine. Secondly, humanistic medicine pertains to what is known as Patient-Centred Medicine (PCM) and other alternatives to PCM, such as narrative-based medicine (NBM) and value-based medicine (VBM). Therefore, PCM is a class of more than one model, whilst the biomedical (BMM) is the only model that pertains to Evidence-Based Medicine (EBM). The main difference is that PCM, in contrast to EBM, focusses on each patient's problems, not just the diagnosis. I chose BPSM as a representative sub-model from the main patient-centred class, since the differences between BPSM and other models within the humanistic approaches are made on various methods of achieving the same goal. The distinctions between disease and suffering and the object versus subject approach contrast the two general classes (evidence-based medicine and value-based medicine/patient-centred medicine).

As conveyed at the beginning of this chapter, conventionally, we refer to the binomial components: the doctor as variable "x" and the patient as variable "*y*." Also, because the definitions for each variable within the model are not clearly stated, as proven previously, I will start from their neutral definitions and add the major components based on the BPSM descriptions. To "*x*," the neutral definition is as follows: a licensed, active medical professional, specialised in a general or specific medical branch, conducts medical examinations, makes diagnoses, prescribes and gives treatments, substance based and/or interventional based (surgical or mechanical) and considers preventive care by applying methods and treatments for specific conditions. And to "*y*," the neutral definition of the patient is an individual afflicted with an illness and/or undergoing treatment for a particular ailment, injury or disorder—see Table 3.1. A schematic representation of the values that the doctor and the patient can ascribe individually or taken together as are in the relationship, based on Kit Fine's Semantic Relationism applied in the medical context—both theoretical and contextual, where *b* is the doctor (Dr. Breuer), whilst *f* and *s* are the patients, Frederic and Sigmund, respectively, from each of the presented cases, C1.1 and C1.2. Descriptions of humanistic medicine (like BPSM) are exhaustive in comparison with those of BMM. For this reason, I selected only a few excerpts that nonetheless serve the aim of this chapter:

> They [humanistic or humane medical practitioners] (...) include the patient's psychological and social dimensions (...) <<to make it [humanized biomedicine] relational, partnership-oriented, individually responsive, and compassionate>> [2, p. 10]

> Instead of the physician being rationally concerned in an emotionally detached manner for the patient's diseased body part, the humanistic or humane practitioner cares both rationally and emotionally for the health of the patient qua person. The underlying value of this type of medical practice is empathy, which shapes a physician's stance. Through this stance, the physician may become aware of the "eidetic" features of a patient's illness, including losses of wholeness, certainty, control, freedom to act, and the familiar world (...). Moreover, the physician recognizes that a patient's mind/body often cures itself and that often the role of both the physician and patient is to assist in that process and not to hinder it. The patient-physician relationship is one of mutual respect, for the role and contribution of each other in the healing process. [2, p. 13]

Henceforth, we can assert that Marcum's perspective—as it was proven for C1.1 and C1.2—reveals that (1) the biomedical model does not necessarily reflect a non-humanistic approach (C1.1), since it depends on the patient's set of beliefs and expectations and (2) the biopsychosocial model does not necessarily imply a humanistic approach, based on empathic care if the patient is pragmatically oriented and does not put value in the humane aspect within the medical encounter but rather to have his medical condition "solved."

In the first case, C1.1, Dr. Breuer and Frederic shared the same conceptual understanding concerning Frederic's medical condition. They were in a tacit, mutual agreement, without differences in opinions, pursuing Frederic's best outcome. Consequently, they had a positive, synergistic interaction. In contrast, in the second case, C 1.2, the doctor and the patient were in a dysfunctional interaction where the patient's best health outcome was not accomplished. Therefore, their interaction was antagonistic. In Kit Fine's semantic relationism terms, this in-depth analysis endorses that "not only which values every single variable can assume, when taken on its own, but also which values several variables can assume when taken together" [3, p. 31]. In other words, when taken together, we acknowledged that variables *b* and *f/s* assumed a positive value when they shared the same intrinsic features, namely, they had the same beliefs (BMM-BMM or BPSM-BPSM approach).

In contrast, their relational value was harmful when they did not share it. This observation underlines the importance of cross-contextuality, meaning that *b* should tend to assume a different external value if the *f/s* does not share the same intrinsic features as *b*—whilst the vice versa does not apply in a patient-centred medical practice. Therefore, the internal values that a physician assumes on their own should be expressed externally, relationally, only if the patient shares the same intrinsic features with the doctor.

Therefore, this analysis brings to light several critical insights regarding medical practice models through the lens of semantic relationism. It reveals that neither the biomedical nor the biopsychosocial model fully accommodates the complexities of the doctor-patient relationship and a one-size-fits-all model is insufficient for patients' diverse needs and values.

In conclusion, this exploration of medical practice models through the prism of semantic relationism reveals significant gaps in how patient care is conceptualised and delivered. On the sense and sensibility that the practice of medicine entails, this chapter advocates for a paradigm shift regarding mentality towards a more flexible, relationship-centred approach that acknowledges the individuality of patient experiences and values.

References

1. Solomon M, Simon JR, Kincaid H (2017) The Routledge companion to philosophy of medicine. Routledge, New York
2. Marcum JA (2008) Humanizing modern medicine. An introductory philosophy of medicine. Springer, Dordrecht. https://doi.org/10.1007/978-1-4020-6797-6
3. Fine K (2007) Semantic relationism. Wiley-Blackwell, New York. https://doi.org/10.1002/9780470690826
4. Sedda A, Manfredi V, Bottini G, Cristani M, Murino V (2012) Automatic human interaction understanding: lessons from a multidisciplinary approach. Front Hum Neurosci 6(57):1–3
5. Ruusuvuori J (2001) Looking means listening: coordinating displays of engagement in doctor–patient interaction. Soc Sci Med 52:1093–1108
6. Cattaneo L, Rizzolatti G (2009) The mirror neuron system. Arch Neurol 66:557–560
7. Rizzolatti G, Craighero L (2004) The mirror-neuron system. Annu Rev Neurosci 27:169–192
8. Ray J (2016) Encyclopedia of personality and individual differences. Springer. https://doi.org/10.1007/978-3-319-28099-8
9. Buccino G, Amore M (2008) Mirror neurons and the understanding of behavioural symptoms in psychiatric disorders. Curr Opin Psychiatry 21:281–285

Chapter 4
Bench and Bedside Medicine: A One-Way Contamination

4.1 Introduction

If we assert that medicine is both science and art, we acknowledge its multifaceted nature. Medicine is a science because of its objectivity derived from rigorous research studies and art because it implies a subjective, human-to-human approach. As such, one must pursue the challenge of integrating objective, scientific knowledge and evidence-based practices with humanistic values like empathy, compassion and creativity in providing comprehensive patient care. This science embodies human values whilst practising according to the latest and generalised scientific discoveries applied to each patient's needs. In recent decades, scholars, including prominent figures like George Engel and James Marcum, have advocated for integrating all aspects that define a patient as a person—not just their biological components—and for the "re-humanization of modern medicine."

Since, from all humanistic disciplines, philosophy plays a central role in understanding medicine's complex dimensions, I will use philosophy as a theoretical tool throughout this work. The intricate relationship between philosophy and medicine has been explored for the past decades, focussing on philosophy's existence, development and implications in/and/for/of medicine [1]. The field of philosophy of medicine developed gradually over time, given the theoretical analysis and explanation of meta-medical issues through concepts like health, disease, illness and suffering, as well as the values and norms underlying medicine as science and practice [1–8]. Scholars delineated the contours of this field by examining the metaphysical, epistemological and ethical dimensions of medicine. Distinct from bioethics, but at the same time, bioethics' foundation, philosophy of medicine addresses epistemological questions about clinical judgement, medical knowledge acquisition methods, metaphysical positions, assumptions, and ontological commitments inherent in the medical worldviews of medical practice models, and ethics considerations linked to the moral foundations of medical practice [2, 3, 6–9].

G.-P. Florea, *Metacognition and Medical Humanities in Medical Education*, New Paradigms in Healthcare, https://doi.org/10.1007/978-3-032-01070-4_4

From epistemological considerations, modern medicine is grounded on empirical, evidence-based aspects from scientific observation, experimentation and analysis. At its foundation lies systematic research through validation, using biomedical knowledge to understand and address health and disease.

The metaphysical considerations involve the mechanical, reductionist view of medicine, which seeks to explain health and disease in terms of mechanistic, deterministic processes governed by physical laws. This view emphasises understanding disease mechanisms, causality and interventions based on linear cause-and-effect relationships. The ontological dimension implies the biological and holistic views of health and disease, highlighting the material and physical properties and their interactions with the environment [1].

On the one hand, mechanical biomedicine explores the human body's structures, functions and processes at molecular, cellular and organismal levels from the biological perspective. On the other hand, holistic biopsychosocial medicine explores the interconnectedness of mind, body, spirit and social environment by integrating biological, psychological, social and spiritual factors to understand and promote well-being. Thus, health and disease are acknowledged within a person's broader context.

Since George Engel proposed a new medical model of disease "for the scientific tasks and social responsibilities" [10, p. 129], the biopsychosocial model, as a solution to the limitations of the traditional biomedical model, has been the subject of significant pondering over reductionist and holistic medicine [11–14]. In this context, the emphasis is on the patient's dehumanisation [1] due to the dichotomy of the human mind and body [15], the reductionist-mechanic view of the person, and the overuse of technology to the detriment of doctor-patient communication, a trademark of the biomedical approach [12, 16–21]. These models relate to the metaphysical differences among disease-illness, health-wellbeing, body-person and object-subject. These conceptual differences have been addressed in medical research and practice due to their acknowledged impact on patient outcomes [22–24].

From a biomedical perspective, health is defined as the absence of disease or "the view of health as the logical opposite of disease" [25, p. 30] and disease as a consequence of a "deviation from the norm of measurable biological (somatic) variables" [10, p. 130]. However, Engel argues that precise definitions of health and disease, or the states of being well and sick, along with their demarcations, are elusive due to the influence of cultural, social and psychological factors [10]. Furthermore, these concepts acquired different values depending on each paradigm that governed medicine throughout history.

Thus, philosophy of medicine reveals the multiple layers on which medicine unfolds based on the complexities of the human condition [10]. It explores the nature of human suffering, meaning, purpose and existence by addressing questions about the deeper existential, philosophical and spiritual dimensions of health, illness and healing [13].

Persistent disputes between theory and practice about how a doctor should approach a patient—reductionist-mechanic or holistic-humanistic, by adopting one model of care over another—highlight the need for a deeper understanding of key concepts used in medical research and care such as theories, models and approaches. Only by examining the meanings behind the words we use can we begin to address this conflict and work towards resolving the issue of dehumanised modern medicine for its rehumanisation.

4.2 Theories

A theory is a set of propositions with explanatory power regarding phenomena. The theory thus provides an illustrative and predictive *model* for that class of phenomena; if new proofs show that the theory is invalidated, then the theory is rejected and changed according to the latest evidence [26]. Also, when the theory is commonly accepted, it becomes a principle (ibid.). It is a conjunction between the theoretical assumptions and derived principles within a research area. Understanding and explaining data is more accessible with the knowledge provided by a theory [27]. Theories imply rules that define certain phenomena through analysis and prediction [28]. In medical epistemology, theories are meant to explain the causes of disease.

When using theory to explain causes, there is a difference between a *medical researcher* (bench medicine) and a *medical practitioner* (bedside medicine). If the former needs to determine a biological cause related to a disease, the latter needs to explain the cause of a symptom by identifying the disease [29]. Consequently, a medical professional who is not a researcher does not inquire about the biological cause of a patient's disease but the cause of the symptom. However, this is not meant to claim that doctors should not be centred on grasping the underlying cause of a patient's disease but to assess a hypothesis by pursuing medical investigations that would justify the possibility of patient *x* having disease *y* or, in other words, to differentiate between disease *y* and disease *w*.

For example the Germ Theory of Disease, considered a fundamental principle in medicine, explains the causality between microbial aetiology of infectious diseases and other diseases based on Henle-Koch's postulates [30]. When clinicians examine patients with symptoms suggesting an infectious disease, they will reach this diagnosis by first assessing the symptoms, running specific tests to identify the infectious agent and then, if necessary, identifying the source. *Stricto* sensu, the causes of those symptoms have already been documented through medical research. Because each class of disease is explained by specific theories belonging to that class,[1] the clinician needs to differentiate between diagnoses by assessing the hypotheses that can justify the symptoms and not by inquiring about what has already been proven through research.

[1] E.g. genetic diseases are explained through genetic theories, immune diseases through immunological ones and so on.

4.3 Models

Models, on the other hand, refer to a pattern from which one can design, imitate or make an analogy over something otherwise difficult to observe or explore [31]. Moreover, models are meant to represent and predict the behaviour of a system, describe the relationship between variables and identify the underlying processes within the system [32]. They are at the core of research based on their intended purpose: qualitative, quantitative or mixed. Nevertheless, the word "model" covers distinct significance depending on the context in which it is used in medicine: (1) related to *research*, it implies "a system of postulates, data, and inferences presented as a mathematical description of an entity or state of affairs" [31] or (2) *conceptual* models used to offer a simplified image of complex ideas or concepts.

A qualitative medical model should be approached according to their usage and purpose, whether in research or clinical practice. In medical studies, their goal slightly differs if referring to quantitative or qualitative research methods. Quantitative research (QnR) contrasts with qualitative research (QlR), because the aim is to bring evidence that would prove or disprove a theory. On the other hand, qualitative medical research aims to describe, comprehend and clarify phenomena [33]. QlR complements QnR research, because it brings findings that explain the phenomena rather than validating or invalidating a hypothesis or theory. QlR describes, decodes and translates natural phenomena, whilst QnR examines trends and rates of recurrence [34]. A qualitative model used in QnR systematically analyses the data collection techniques or the design employed within the study [32]. A qualitative model applied in QlR focusses on examining data collection techniques of interviews, focus groups or any other qualitative methods of inquiry used [35, 36].

Qualitative studies in medicine focus on how individuals comprehend and assign significance to their personal experiences (phenomenological approach) and examine the cultural and social elements of a particular group, including their historical, religious, economic, political and environmental aspects (ethnographical approach), or explores the social processes that occur during human interactions within a medical setting, a grounded theory approach [34, 37].

New theories may be developed in both types of research based on various methods. In QlR, new theories can result once the data is systematically gathered and analysed through comparative analysis by coding and categorising it to identify patterns and concepts through the grounded theory method [38–40]. Therefore, the phenomenon under study is explained through the theory or theories that emerge from the processed data. Quantitative studies can either support or challenge existing theories. However, the results of QnR may not only refine or modify the theory being assessed but may also lead, in some cases, to the development of new ones [32].

Thus, whilst the primary purpose of qualitative research (QlR) is to explain phenomena by generating hypotheses and theories that emerge from collected and analysed data, the primary goal of quantitative research (QnR) is to evaluate hypotheses and theories, and only as a result of the gathered evidence, to develop new theories.

QlR seeks to develop an understanding of social phenomena in natural settings by emphasising participants' values, experiences and interpretations of the subject being explored: "beliefs and understandings, people's lived experience" [34, p. 12]. It explores, narrates and explains phenomena, primarily focussing on processes of human behaviour: "Qualitative research helps to understand the patterns of health behaviours, describe illness experiences, design health interventions, and develop healthcare theories" [41, p. 6].

Before going further, it is essential to stress the distinction that Barbour [33] makes between "evidence" and "findings" in the way that the latter explicitly attributes agency to the researcher in contrast to the former, which highlights the significance of the context in which data is produced, understood and communicated. Hence, the results brought by QnR are evidence, whilst those by QlR are findings.

Suppose we start from the premise that models are theoretical constructs that offer an idealised simplified representation of a system or phenomenon. In this case, we are referring to two major classes of models that concern medical knowledge: dualistic and holistic, reductionist and emergentist, and biological and biopsychosocial [1, p. 8]. Each research medical model has been extended to new variants that differentiate themselves through the multifaceted perspectives they bring to the same aspect. For example the traditional research model has been solely linked to the biological element of addressing a disease without acknowledging a person's psychological and social traits. The biopsychosocial inquiry model evolved as an extension of the traditional research model [10]. Later, new variants of the biopsychosocial model were introduced, for example the biopsychosocial-spiritual model [18] and the biopsychosocial-digital model [42].

As Hewa and Hetherington [43] underlined, medical research models rely on specific conceptual theories. The biomedical is explained through Max Weber's rationalised theory,[2] whilst the biopsychosocial model is through Ludwig von Bertalanffy's General System Theory.[3] The former model is mechanistic, following "calculability, predictability, and control". At the same time, the latter is focussed on "the general quality of life, clean environment, and psychological, or spiritual stability of life" [43, p. 129].

BMM is grounded on numerical data—evidence-based medicine—whilst BPSM is grounded on a mixed method of research using numerical and non-numerical data analysis through qualitative studies. Considering BPSM's principles in addressing the psychological and social dimensions of disease and the biological dimensions, Engel brought qualitative indicators through the patient's experience of disease, illness and suffering. Due to its focus on quality rather than quantity, BPSM of research is thus oriented towards research findings and not research evidence, as opposed to BMM, which is quantitative.

---

[2]The industrialised modern society is no longer based on values, traditions and emotions but on reason and rationality [66, 67].

[3]A general theory can explain systems in all scientific domains [68].

The biopsychosocial model has its drawbacks, including the complexity of its multifactorial features and perspectives, alongside a lack of clear definition. Measuring these parameters is a challenging task, because there is a limitation in the amount of evidence-based research available for BPSM, as it cannot be widely assessed or validated. Its implementation may also be biased towards certain factors or perspectives, potentially favouring some over others [44]. BPSM is a model without a method [45] in contrast to biomedicine, which has a mature and empirically validated work-frame. All the critiques regarding biopsychosocial medicine underline how unstable and unreliable it is as a research model.

On the one hand, it is worth noting that BPSM can offer insights that BMM cannot: a holistic understanding of the patient rather than just the disease by focussing on the patient as a whole [12]. Because the multidisciplinary framework ensures a comprehensive approach to treatment with the potential to improve patient-centred medicine, its complexity and lack of clarity pose challenges during implementation.

On the other hand, BMM has played a crucial role in expanding medical knowledge and treatments regardless of its disease-centred rather than patient-centred framework.

4.3.1 Models in Medical Practice

In medical practice, a "qualitative" model can facilitate the implementation of evidence derived from quantitative research (QnR) or findings obtained from qualitative research (QlR) [33]. At the same time, a research model may provide guidelines on approaching, assessing, diagnosing and therapeutically treating a patient. In this context, models are abstract representations derived from both types of research. In other words, a research model becomes the source and resource of a model of medical practice. From this perspective, we can assert that these abstract representations have the potential to influence the medical practitioner on a spectrum ranging from (1) the personal set of beliefs that shape the decision-making process (e.g., the physician's view of health, disease, illness, and the patient—whether reduced to their parts or regarded as a whole) to, as a consequence, (2) the physician's behaviour in the doctor-patient approach. The biomedical and biopsychosocial models in medical practice are extensions of the biomedical and biopsychosocial paradigms of inquiry in medical research [10]. Furthermore, a medical professional's beliefs, shaped by formal medical education and research, inevitably manifest in doctor-patient interactions and relationships.

According to Lucchiari et al. [46], physicians follow "mindlines," a blend of analytic and intuitive thinking, which differs from decision making based on guidelines. They assert that physicians' minds work on a cognitive framework, integrating and providing meaning to the flow of data from the environment, such as patients' symptoms and clinical tests, naming it a "mental model" [46, p. 290]. Derived from this model, they provide a work frame that balances analytic and intuitive mental processing based on knowledge and experience, avoiding biased heuristic thinking—a "cognitive balanced model" (ibid.). In a more complex understanding of a mental model, Holtrop et al. [47] propose this concept as a solution to translating and implementing science, starting from the fact that "mental models are comprised of interrelated memories, conceptual knowledge, and causal beliefs that create an understanding of how something works in the real world and forms expectations about future events" [47, p. 2]. Also, they acknowledge that each patient has a mental model on their own of how the medical encounter would take place, based on their previous experience or through "the transfer of cultural knowledge through media and social networks" [ibid.]. Based on the patient's mental model, their perspective will determine how they will address questions or express their beliefs to obtain the desired investigations and therapeutic strategies from the physician or comply with those presented by the doctor without cooperation in the sense of shared decision-making. Conversely, due to their mental model lenses, the doctor decides whether to accept or not the information and changes given by the patient. From this perspective, it is worth noting the emphasis on how the understanding of one's mental model can shape one's behaviour in each situation and how this can be pivotal in "understanding, anticipating, and overcoming implementation challenges" [ibid.] for evidence-based interventions.

An extended optic of the mental model type is the shared mental model (SMM), built by Floren et al. [48], where "an individually held, organized, cognitive representation of and/or team-related knowledge that is held in common among healthcare providers who must interact as a team in pursuit of common objectives for patient care" [48, p. 16] is essential for efficient and productive decision-making in healthcare teamwork. However, the validity of this model is uncertain [49]—the problem relates to the medical team members' beliefs and how they may impact their collaborative work.[4]

Therefore, research models and care models that involve the distinct mental models of both the doctor and the patient are not the same, although models of care frequently derive from research. This fact reveals the complexity between research-derived frameworks and practical care models: whilst research models inform the unique mental models of each participant, these mental models, in turn, deeply influence the care models applied in doctor-patient interactions. These mental models reflect individual cognitive frameworks, beliefs and expectations, which can diverge significantly despite being influenced by overarching research-based models.

[4] Consequently, in Chap. 3 A Semantic Relationism Approach to Doctor-Patient Relationship, I argue that models related to the mental dimension can be classified into intrinsic and extrinsic cognitive features, which apply to both the patient and the physician in the clinical context.

4.3.2 Models of Care

In *The Oath* and *The Law* chapters, the Hippocratic Corpus offers information regarding medical education and apparel [50]. Only in the past half-century have debates in the philosophy of medicine emerged, questioning how medical professionals perceive or understand the concepts of illness and disease, as well as the patient as both an object (body) and a subject (person) [1]. Scholars are trying to underline the need to understand patients' unicity and set different paradigms or models by distinguishing between mechanistic and holistic aspects associated with humanistic medical knowledge and practice [17, 19, 51–53]. The leading figure attributed to the humanistic model derives from the biopsychosocial theory set by George Engel [10]. Since then, prominent authors have endorsed it [10, 12, 19, 54–57].

James Marcum distinguishes between biomedical and biopsychosocial models of care by the metaphysical positions, presuppositions and ontological commitments each of the two models ascribes [1]. He asserts that modern medicine derives from Western culture and that medical practitioners assign a particular metaphysical position or stance—monism, dualism or holism—in their relationship with a patient according to the worldview they, the physicians, choose mechanistic and/or holistic. In contrast, in his highly cited article, Davis-Floyd [58] describes three healthcare models: (1) the technocratic, (2) humanistic and (3) holistic, where technocratic medicine is "high tech/low touch," humanistic medicine is "high tech/high touch," and holistic[5] is "low tech/high touch" [58, p. S19].

Similarly to Maare E. Tamm [13], Marcum classifies models based on their focus on medical professionals who acknowledge this metaphysical stance as humane practitioners [1]. Therefore, it conceptually transformed Engel's biopsychosocial research model into a humanistic model, implying that it encompasses the holistic understanding of the human body and the approach that derives from its implementation in the medical practice, "the compassionate model of care."

Moreover, according to Marcum, humanistic models are grounded in "an ontological commitment to organicism," which is reflected in the view of the patient as an integrative system, serving as both an etiological and therapeutic marker of disease [1, p. 29]. By *organicism,* he refers to organismal wholes rather than mere compositional parts. He asserts that the biomedical model is reductionist and materialist, whilst the humanistic model is emergentist and organicist, a fundamental difference in their approaches. The biomedical model operates through a bottom-up process, whereas the humanistic model employs a top-down perspective [1, p. 31]. Furthermore, Marcum argues that the two models lack a shared conceptual foundation, which is why proponents of the humanistic model view it as *supervening* the biomedical one.

---

[5] David-Floyd defines the holistic model of medicine as the complementary branch of medicine which encompasses "hands-on energy, nutritional medicine, herbal therapies" [58] focussed on natural healing methods where technology may be an add-on.

Furthermore, Marcum questions the possibility of a paradigm shift from the biomedical to the humane medical model. He compares the two models based on how each approaches the mind-body problem: dualistic for BMM, where the doctor is a technician reducing the patient to the physical elements that compose their body, and holistic for BPSM, where the doctor is a humane practitioner that acknowledges the person's body as well as their mind [1, p. 11–12]. In response to this contested argument—and paradoxically in support of the holistic view via biomedicine—the answer may be found in psycho-neuro-endocrine-immunology (PNEI) and personalised medicine (PM)– as explained in Chap. 5, Should Mentality Overpass Paradigms in Medicine?. The reason is the shared premise on which they ground their theory: individual differences in a person's physiological, psychological, social and environmental factors (or epigenetic) that determine or influence the development of one or multiple diseases. PNEI studies how the nervous, endocrine and immune systems interact with a person's psychological traits [59–61]. At the same time, PM is an approach to medical treatment that considers individual variability in genes, environment and lifestyle based on which medical decisions and possible therapeutics are tailored to the individual patient [62].

Therefore, for each of these two, PNEI and PM, at the centre is not the concept of disease per se but the physiological and psychological characteristics that make up a person's unique clinical picture based on which the desired outcome is specific to that patient and not on the general population, under the statistical significance indicator. The question that inherently arises from these two is on which grounds are they based, from a philosophical perspective? Their inquiry is both a bottom-up and top-down process, since they search for the biological makeup or changes in a disease—PM is genome-centred in correlation with epigenetics. At the same time, PNEI is linked with "epigenetic effects, endogenous influences, environmental factors, and microbiome differences" [63, p. 473]. On the other hand, personalised medicine is not person centred if the psychological and social context is not addressed in the populational framework and, vice versa, health within a population cannot be understood and conceived without knowing the individuals who are part of that population [64, p. 78].

4.4 Approaches

In medical *research*, "approach" refers to the methodologies and strategies employed to advance medical knowledge, such as clinical trials, epidemiological studies, basic science and translational research.

The *clinical* approach refers to the systematic way healthcare professionals assess, diagnose and treat patients: the initial patient evaluation, the gathering of medical history, physical examination, the ordering and interpretation of diagnostic tests and the formulation of a treatment plan. The clinical approach is guided by evidence-based practices and tailored to each patient's individual needs: it focusses on the treatment modalities used to manage or treat diseases with a wide range of interventions, including pharmacological treatments, physical therapies, surgical interventions and alternative or complementary therapies. The therapeutic "approach" is multidisciplinary—various healthcare specialists collaborate for the best patient outcomes. The preventive "approach" implies actions that need to be pursued to prevent the occurrence of disease or mitigate its impact: vaccinations, screening programmes, lifestyle modifications and public health initiatives.

There is also the patient-centred "approach," meaning that the medical professional focusses on patients' preferences, needs and values in all aspects of their care.

The ethical and legal "approach" focusses on the implications of ethical principles and legal requirements in medical practice—patient consent, confidentiality, end-of-life care, equity in healthcare, etc.

4.5 The Theory, Model and Approach Conjunction in Medicine

As proven so far, the terms "theory," "model" and "approach" have multiple and distinct meanings. Each contributes to the understanding of medical research and the application of medical knowledge in medical practice.

Since theory is an explanation supported by evidence concerning aspects of the natural world, it provides a framework for understanding observations and making predictions about future events or discoveries. In medicine, theories might explain diseases' underlying mechanisms, genetic factors' impact on health or the body's response to treatments. They are supported by empirical evidence and are often commonly accepted within the scientific community. However, theories may evolve as new evidence emerges, meaning they are not static. For example since the Germ Theory of Disease was postulated, diseases caused by infectious agents are treatable thanks to the research and treatment strategies that evolved from this theory.

In medicine, physical, mathematical or conceptual models play a significant role in understanding complex systems, predicting outcomes, and exploring the potential effects of interventions. As previously mentioned, a model in medicine is a representation or simulation of a biological process, disease or treatment. In addition, models are often used to test hypotheses or design experiments. Whilst they are based on existing knowledge and evidence, models simplify reality and focus on particular aspects of a system, which can sometimes limit their applicability. For example the biopsychosocial model of health and disease may be considered a conceptual model that integrates biological, psychological and social factors to understand patient health and guide treatment; thus, it is more complex than the other conceptual model, the simpler mechanistic biomedical one.

An approach in medicine refers to a specific method or strategy used in diagnosing, treating or managing patients. Approaches are practical in nature and informed by theories and models, but they focus on applying medical knowledge in clinical settings. They are actionable and tailored to specific circumstances or conditions.

Also, since they are often described in terms of protocols, techniques or care philosophies, medical approaches may vary depending on the medical speciality, patient needs and available resources.

In summary, theories provide broad explanations based on the evidence related to the natural world; models offer simplified, conceptual representations to understand complex biological systems or predict outcomes; medical approaches describe specific methods or strategies applied in clinical practice. These delineations, therefore, prove their particular role in advancing medical science and improving patient care. Nevertheless, the confusion between models of health and disease and approaches in medical care occurs, because they are misleadingly used interchangeably and prone to practice biases in medical care. One of the significant causes resides in the conceptual transference from medical research to patient care.

4.6 Conceptual Transference from Medical Research to Patient Care

As the argument built in the last sections, medical research models offer biological evidence of disease and focus on explaining the cause of a symptom in BMM. In BPSM, models focus on the framework of the interplay among the biological, psychological and social factors that can explain the underlying mechanisms of illness and well-being, addressing the mind-body gap.

Applied to medical practice, the BMM is considered a "popular or folk model of disease" [10, p. 130]. At the same time, the BPSM is a *humanistic* model of disease adopted by medical practitioners according to how they approach a patient as a person, in contrast to BMM, which approaches the patient as a machine [1, p. 11]. Therefore, they are not scientific models but conceptual or personal beliefs [10, p. 130] expressed indirectly in their interaction with the patient. Following Holtrop's [47] argumentation as presented above, I argued that they may fall into the abstract categorisation of the mental model subclass, derived from a translation and implementation of methods of inquiry into doctor-patient interaction. Accordingly, they can be interpreted as unconscious, thus, implicit mental models that doctors use in their relationships with patients. This "contamination" may come from various lines, especially from medical education, the predefined clinical protocols that shape a doctor's thinking in a specific frame in conjunction with each doctor's belief system. These mental attitudes and predispositions are then transferred in the doctor-patient interaction.

> The biomedical model was devised by medical scientists for the study of disease. As such it was a scientific model; that is, it involved a shared set of assumptions and rules of conduct based on the scientific method and constituted a blueprint for research. Not all models are scientific. Indeed, broadly defined, a model is nothing more than a belief system utilized to explain natural phenomena, to make sense out of what is puzzling or disturbing. [10, p. 130]

Marcum [1, 65] classifies models of medical care according to their metaphysical presupposition and ontological commitment. Because the BMM is disease centred, it falls under the metaphysical presumption of reductionism and the ontological commitment to physicalism. On the other hand, because the BPSM focusses on the patient's psychological and social dimensions, it is thus committed to ontological organicism. These lines of approaching health and disease or illness determine a "predisposition" towards a specific frame of inquiry and understanding of health and disease. These biomedical and biopsychosocial predispositions of understanding health and disease, well-being, illness and suffering have been transferred from medical research to medical practice, impacting the physicians' way of approaching patients.

Consequently, a biomedical, reductionist and biopsychosocial model emerged, the so-called humanist [1]. It is what Engel named "folk models" constituted by "culturally derived belief systems about disease (…), but they are not scientific models" [10, p. 130]. Since biomedicine's principles were transferred from the bench (research) to the patient's bedside, it significantly impacted the doctor-patient relationship. It "contaminated" the perspective-taking in choosing a model of inquiring about health and disease or illness from research to medical practice; it determined doctors to adhere to one of the medical research principles, hence transforming a research model to a doctor-patient relationship *folk* model that relies on the doctor's belief system. Doctors may thus be prone to adopting beliefs aligned with research principles embedded in medical education and clinical protocols. Henceforth, a physician working under the biomedical precepts is focussed on disease, and the one working under the biopsychosocial principles is focussed on the patient's biological determinants and their experience in the process. Therefore, a conflict between beliefs embedded in the doctor's and the patient's mental models may occur. This phenomenon can be considered conceptual contamination from bench to bedside medicine.

Moreover, medical professionals who require improvement in transferrable skills like empathy and compassion are considered to belong to the category that adheres to the biomedical model of care. In contrast, those following the BPSM model of care, also known as holistic, have a compassionate and empathetic approach, assimilated with a humanistic approach to their interaction with the patient [1]. Consequently, a categorisation of doctor-patient interaction based on a doctor's set of beliefs as a reductionist, mechanic or holistic, therefore, a humanised model of care derived, according to Marcum's writings. Employing semantic relationism theory, doctors choose one of the alleged models according to their set of beliefs—whether they accept or not to assess the existence of other dimensions besides the biological, such as a patient's psychological and social extents, as argued in Chap. 3 A Semantic Relationism Approach to Doctor-Patient Relationship.

4.7 Conclusion

A researcher adopting a specific work frame is essential in pursuing that particular line of inquiry, since they would be otherwise unable to have a purpose-driven goal and a working frame of investigation. If this predisposition is mandatory for a researcher, a medical professional's explicit adherence to one of the folk models derived from research principles may be inadequate, since it is not always compatible with the patient's set of beliefs. Hence, a doctor's imposition of their health-disease set of beliefs may bring tensions in the doctor-patient relationship and negatively affect the patient's compliance with the treatment and, implicitly, the disease's outcome.

This contamination from medical research to practice made the words "model" and "approach" wrongly overlap and used interchangeably according to the world-views adopted by each of them—BMM research models overlapping with an approach related to BMM's worldview and BPSM research model overlapping with an approach associated with BPSM's worldview. These overlaps determined various medical care approaches and created a false dichotomy between reductionist and holistic medicine or mechanic and humanistic care. Why a false dichotomy? Because the body's architecture and function can be explained mechanistically, whilst the person, for example the patient, is a whole entity, mechanically, whilst manifesting into the world as a mind-body unity with all its complexities that encompass it. To have doctors split into categories related to types of approaching patients according to research models kills the art of medicine, reducing it to a theory and creating, ultimately, the ambiguity of what human life, a patient as a person, really is.

References

1. Marcum JA (2008) An introductory philosophy of medicine. Humanizing modern medicine. Springer. https://doi.org/10.1007/978-1-4020-6797-6
2. Schramme T, Edwards S (2017) Handbook of the philosophy of medicine. Springer, Dordrecht
3. Pellegrino ED (1986) Philosophy of medicine: towards a definition. J Med Philos 11:9–16
4. Stempsey WE (2005) The philosophy of medicine: development of a discipline. Med Health Care Philos 7:243–251
5. Fenton R (2018) What is the place for philosophy within the field of medicine? A review of contemporary issues in medical ethics. Philos Ethics Humanit Med 13:1–5
6. Pellegrino ED (1998) What the philosophy of medicine is. Theor Med Bioeth 19:315–336
7. Pellegrino ED (2006) Toward a reconstruction of medical morality. Am J Bioeth 6:65–71
8. Pellegrino ED, Thomasma DC (1993) The virtues in medical practice. Oxford University Press
9. Sadegh-Zadeh K (2015) Handbook of analytic philosophy of medicine. Springer, Dordrecht. https://doi.org/10.1007/978-94-017-9579-1
10. Engel GL (1977) The need for a new medical model: a challenge for biomedicine. Science 196:129–136

11. Cormack B, Stilwell P, Coninx S, Gibson J (2022) The biopsychosocial model is lost in translation: from misrepresentation to an enactive modernization. Physiother Theory Pract 39(11):2273–2288. https://doi.org/10.1080/09593985.2022.2080130
12. Wade DT, Halligan PW (2017) The biopsychosocial model of illness: a model whose time has come. Clin Rehabil 31:995–1004
13. Tamm ME (1993) Models of health and disease. Br J Med Psychol 66:213–228
14. Tauber AI (2017) Medical humanism. Part 1: Philosophical and historical underpinnings. In: Marcum JA (ed) The Bloomsbury companion to contemporary philosophy of medicine. Bloomsbury Academic, London, pp 161–182
15. Bottaccioli F (2014) La fine della grande illusione del riduzionismo in biologia e in medicina. Epistemologia 2014:5–21
16. Boyle J, Morriss J (1979) The crisis in medicine: models, myths, and metaphors. Et Cetera 36:261–274
17. Marcum JA (2017) The "new" medical model, fragmented clinical care and philosophy of medicine. Can Med Assoc J 189:E897
18. Saad M, de Medeiros R, Mosini AC (2017) Are we ready for a true biopsychosocial–spiritual model? the many meanings of "spiritual". Medicines 4:79
19. Fuller J (2017) The new medical model: a renewed challenge for biomedicine. Can Med Assoc J 189:E640–E641
20. Wieten S (2018) Expertise in evidence-based medicine: a tale of three models. Philos Ethics Humanit Med 13:2
21. Duncan G (2000) Mind-body dualism and the biopsychosocial model of pain: what did Descartes really say? J Med Philos 25:485–513
22. Benedetti F (2009) Placebo effects. Understanding the mechanisms in health and disease. Oxford University Press
23. Benedetti F (2013) Placebo and the new physiology of the doctor-patient relationship. Physiol Rev 93:1207–1246
24. Evers AWM, Colloca L, Blease C et al (2018) Implications of placebo and nocebo effects for clinical practice: expert consensus. Psychother Psychosom 87:204–210
25. Engelhardt HT, Spicker SF (1975) Evaluation and explanation in the biomedical sciences. Trans-disciplinary Symposium on Philosophy and Medicine, I st, Galveston, 1974. https://doi.org/10.1007/978-94-010-1769-5
26. Venes D (2017) Taber's cyclopedic medical dictionary, 23rd edn. F.A. Davis Company, Philadelphia
27. Klein KJ, Zedeck S (2004) Introduction to the special section on theoretical models and conceptual analyses: theory in applied psychology: lessons (re)learned. J Appl Psychol 89:931–933
28. Bates MJ (2005) An introduction to metatheories, theories, and models. In: Fisher KE, Erdelez S, McKechnie L (eds) Theories of information behavior. American Society for Information Science and Technology, pp 1–24
29. Thagard P (2005) What is a medical theory? In: Paton R, McNamara L (eds) Studies in multidisciplinarity. Elsevier, pp 47–62
30. Evans AS (1978) Causation and disease: a chronological journey: the Thomas Parran lecture. Am J Epidemiol 108:249–258
31. Merriam-Webster.com Dictionary. s.v. "model." In: Definition & meaning—Merriam-Webster. 2023; https://www.merriam-webster.com/dictionary/model. Accessed 11 May 2023
32. Cobelli C, Carson E (2019) Introduction to modeling in physiology and medicine, 2nd edn. Elsevier Academic Press
33. Barbour RS (2000) The role of qualitative research in broadening the 'evidence base' for clinical practice. J Eval Clin Pract 6:155–163
34. Al-Busaidi ZQ (2008) Qualitative research and its uses in health care. Sultan Qaboos Univ Med J 8:11–19
35. Fawcett J (2016) Applying conceptual models of nursing. Springer. https://doi.org/10.1891/9780826180063

36. Neuman B, Fawcett J (2010) The Neuman systems model, 5th edn. Pearson, Upper Saddle River
37. Tavakol M, Torabi S, Zeinaloo AA (2006) Grounded theory in medical education research. Med Educ Online 11:4607
38. Glasser BG, Strauss A (1967) The discovery of grounded theory: strategies for qualitative research. Aldine Transaction, Chicago
39. Noble H, Mitchell G (2016) What is grounded theory? Evid Based Nurs 19:34–35
40. Tie YC, Birks M, Francis K (2019) Grounded theory research: a design framework for novice researchers. SAGE Open Med 7:1–8
41. Renjith V, Yesodharan R, Noronha J, Ladd E, George A (2021) Qualitative methods in health care research. Int J Prev Med. https://doi.org/10.4103/IJPVM.IJPVM_321_19
42. Ahmadvand A, Gatchel R, Brownstein J, Nissen L (2018) The biopsychosocial-digital approach to health and disease: call for a paradigm expansion. J Med Internet Res. https://doi.org/10.2196/JMIR.9732
43. Hewa S, Hetherington RW (1995) Specialists without spirit: limitations of the mechanistic biomedical model. Theor Med 16:129–139
44. Epstein RM, Borrell-Carrio F (2005) The biopsychosocial model: exploring six impossible things. Fam Syst Health 23:426–431
45. Card AJ (2022) The biopsychosociotechnical model: a systems-based framework for human-centered health improvement. Health Syst 12(4):387–407
46. Lucchiari C, Folgieri R, Pravettoni G (2014) Fuzzy cognitive maps: a tool to improve diagnostic decisions. Diagnosi 1:289–293
47. Holtrop JS, Scherer LD, Matlock DD, Glasgow RE, Green LA (2021) The importance of mental models in implementation science. Front Public Health 9:916
48. Floren LC, Donesky D, Whitaker E, Irby DM, ten Cate O, O'Brien BC (2018) Are we on the same page? Shared mental models to support clinical teamwork among health professions learners. Acad Med. https://doi.org/10.1097/ACM.0000000000002019
49. Gisick LM, Webster KL, Keebler JR, Lazzara EH, Fouquet S, Fletcher K, Fagerlund A, Lew V, Chan R (2018) Measuring shared mental models in healthcare. J Patient Saf Risk Manag 23:207–219
50. Hippocrates (2015) The complete works of Hippocrates. Delphi Classics
51. Huda AS (2019) The medical model in mental health. Oxford University Press, Oxford. https://doi.org/10.1093/MED/9780198807254.001.0001
52. Wang X, Hu Y, Tao J, Hu F, Li P, Shao D, Pan HF, Xu T (2021) Design and initial validation of a humanistic care evaluation tool. J Multidiscip Healthc 14:2307–2313
53. Maheux B, Beaudoin C, Berkson L, Côté L, Des Marchais J, Jean P (2000) Medical faculty as humanistic physicians and teachers: the perceptions of students at innovative and traditional medical schools. Med Educ 34:630–634
54. van Schalkwyk G, Diaz E, Rohrbaugh R (2016) The biopsychosocial formulation. In: International medical graduate physicians. Springer, Cham, pp 101–113
55. Borrell-Carrio F, Suchman A, Epstein R (2004) The biopsychosocial model 25 years later: principles, practice, and scientific inquiry. Ann Fam Med 2:576–582
56. Souza PP, Romão AS, Rosa-e-Silva JC, Candido dos Reis F, Nogueira AA, Poli-Neto OB (2011) Qualitative research as the basis for a biopsychosocial approach to women with chronic pelvic pain. J Psychosom Obstet Gynaecol 32:165–172
57. Geraghty KJ, Blease C (2019) Myalgic encephalomyelitis/chronic fatigue syndrome and the biopsychosocial model: a review of patient harm and distress in the medical encounter. Disabil Rehabil 41:3092–3102
58. Davis-Floyd R (2001) The technocratic, humanistic, and holistic paradigms of childbirth. Int J Gynecol Obstet 75:S5–S23
59. Ader R (2007) Psychoneuroimmunology. Elsevier Academic Press, IV
60. Irwin MR (2008) Human psychoneuroimmunology: 20 years of discovery. Brain Behav Immun 22:129–139
61. Daruna JH (2012) Introduction to psychoneuroimmunology, 2nd edn. Elsevier

62. Delpierre C, Lefèvre T (2023) Precision and personalized medicine: what their current definition says and silences about the model of health they promote. Implication for the development of personalized health. Front Sociol 8:1–5
63. Nebert DW, Zhang G (2019) Pharmacogenomics. In: Emery and Rimoin's principles and practice of medical genetics and genomics: foundations. Academic, pp 445–486
64. Giroux É (2020) Is personalized medicine humanist? Arch Philos 83:59–82
65. Marcum JA (2008) Reflections on humanizing biomedicine. Perspect Biol Med 51:392–405
66. Weber M (2005) The Protestant ethic and the spirit of capitalism. Routledge
67. Kalberg S (1980) Max Weber's types of rationality: cornerstones for the analysis of rationalization processes in history. Am J Sociol 85:1145–1179
68. von Bertalanffy L (1968) General system theory: foundations, development, applications. George Braziller

Chapter 5
Should Mentality Overpass Paradigms in Medicine?

5.1 Introduction

Similar to the history of physical optics,[1] medicine transitioned from one way of understanding the human body to another. As shown in the history of medicine, the concepts of health and disease were initially associated with the Hippocratic four humours theory, to which Galen adhered. However, medicine eventually contradicted this view, starting from the premise that the body must be reduced to its parts to understand the whole. Until later discoveries, the four humours theory was the working theory of those times. When it was first coined in the twentieth century, biomedicine emerged from discovering that infectious agents cause specific diseases, creating the connection between biological processes and diseases. It was related only to the research part of medicine and not to the clinical practice [1]. In more recent developments, the understanding of the disease has evolved due to the recognition of the interconnections amongst psychology and neurological, immune, and endocrine systems, as will be elaborated upon subsequently.

Disease is generally understood as a deviation from biological norms identified through measurable abnormalities in body functions or structure. It is the aspect of health that can be directly linked to pathophysiological processes, where Engel critiques the biomedical model for its narrow focus on this dimension alone. Illness refers to the personal experience of symptoms and suffering that is not always directly correlated with the presence of a disease—how the individual perceives and lives with a medical condition, including psychological distress and the impact on their quality of life; Engel's model emphasises the importance of understanding

[1]According to Newton, light was "material corpuscles," in the nineteenth century, "a transverse wave motion," whilst since the beginning of the twentieth century, "light is photons" [2, p. 13].

G.-P. Florea, *Metacognition and Medical Humanities in Medical Education*, New Paradigms in Healthcare, https://doi.org/10.1007/978-3-032-01070-4_5

illness from the patient's perspective by taking into consideration psychological factors and subjective experiences into medical care.

On the other hand, suffering is understood as the impact of disease or illness on an individual's life at a broader existential and emotional level: psychological and emotional responses to both disease symptoms and the social implications of being ill. Engel's approach suggests that suffering is influenced by a broader range of factors beyond the biological, such as the psychological and social. From this standpoint, Engel argues for a holistic approach to healthcare, because biological abnormalities (disease), personal experiences and perceptions (illness), and the broader existential impacts (suffering) are relevant in diagnosis, treatment and care.

Thomas Kuhn [2] defined a paradigm as a shared set of assumptions, concepts, values and practices that guide scientific research within a particular community at a given time. He argued that paradigms can shape how scientists approach problems and questions and claimed that new paradigms can replace old ones through scientific revolution and that two paradigms can coexist. Kuhn tied paradigms to "normal science" and "universally recognised scientific achievements that for a time provide model problems and solutions to a community of practitioners" [2, p. viii]. These accomplishments are distinguished by (1) their novelty, which attracts a committed group of followers away from alternative scientific pursuits, and (2) their openness, which presents a range of unresolved issues for the community of practitioners to address [ibid.]. Kuhn further observed that instances of scientific practice could give rise to specific, coherent traditions of scientific research [2, p. 10]. He also noted the possibility, albeit infrequent, for two paradigms to coexist peacefully in a later "post-paradigm" stage. I shall henceforth refer to achievements that share these two characteristics as paradigms related closely to "normal science."

The possibility of a paradigm shift in modern medicine has been debated on several grounds with a wide range of considerations, from research [3, 4] to health management and care [5–8], clinical decision making [9] and medical education [10–12].

Throughout medicine's history, the theories that explain health and disease have changed from one era to another. Significant historical shifts of understanding, which dictated not only possible definitions of health and disease but also how medical professionals should approach the ill in diagnosing or curing, have been the basis of these changes. Although the concepts of paradigm, theory, model and approach have different meanings, they are often used interchangeably.

5.2 The First Paradigm Shift in Medicine: From the "Divine" to the "Natural Forces" Paradigm

In classical antiquity, between the eighth and sixth centuries BC, *Asklepios* was initially considered an "excellent healer" [13, p. 69] and later as a Graeco-Roman God invoked by the ill [13–15]. After his death, some writings claimed that his "medical arts" related to the god Apollo, Asklepios, being deified and referred to since then as the God of Medicine [16]. Inherently, a cult under his name rose in the fifth century BC [13, p. 70], and many of his adepts followed Asklepios' guiding rules. It is also considered that Asklepios' knowledge was lost for five centuries and that Hippocrates rediscovered it when the worship of Asklepios continued to take place [17, p. xx].

The entire body of knowledge attributed to the Father of Western Medicine, Hippocrates, covers over 60 writings on medical knowledge and practice, known as the *Hippocratic Corpus*, including the Hippocratic oath. Although there is still debate about whether Hippocrates wrote it, the writings align with Hippocrates' theory. The disputed subject of authorship is given by the contradictory information presented, based on two medical philosophies grounded in the schools of thought belonging to Empedocles in Agrigentum and Alcmaeon in Croton [18, p. 9]. The difference between the two resides in the attraction and/or repulsion of the elements considered to form the Universe—Empedocles' view—such as earth, water, air and fire, and that health is maintained through a balance between "moist and dry, cold and hot, bitter and sweet"—Alcmaeon's view [ibid.]. Consequently, the connection between the body and the environment was acknowledged. Furthermore, Plato links the necessity of "understanding the nature of the whole" in medicine and the nature of one's soul (Pl. *Phdr.* 270c), which is underlined in Hippocrates' writing.

Hippocrates profoundly influenced the setting, setting the ground for an objective and objectifiable manner of treating the ill. He describes what we now know as epilepsy in the following terms: "[i]t appears to me to be nowise more divine nor more sacred than other diseases but has a natural cause from the originates like other affections", as underlined in *On the sacred disease* [18, p. 345]. Thus, the Hippocratic Corpus acknowledged that the root cause of disease was not divine but the effect of a natural force. This disease view was one of the critical breakthroughs of medicine at that time.

In addition, Plato emphasised the mind's non-material and immortal nature. At the same time, Aristotle, "the father of logic" and a proponent of the scientific method, pleaded for nature and human life to be grounded in scientific inquiry and explained through causal relationships [19, p. 216]. Consequently, Greek medicine was significantly shaped by these philosophical underpinnings. It moved away from the religious, spiritual perspective on the human medical condition that existed before Hippocrates. This philosophy was characterised by rationality and logic compared to prior understandings of health and disease. In addition, it contributed to developing a dualistic worldview, distinguishing spirit from matter and mind from body.

Before Hippocrates, a physician was both a philosopher and a priest, and the definition of disease consisted of divine input "sent by the divine" [14, p. 425]. Starting with Hippocrates, the physician was no longer a priest but an observer.

Therefore, we can assert that, in the evolutionary steps of medicine, era represents the shift from a mystifying understanding of the human body to a more systematic approach. These theories focussed on (1) disease as a natural process in contrast with Asklepios' view regarding the supernatural forces or punishment from the gods; (2) the need for clinical observation—observing symptoms and disease's progression that would dictate the type of treatment; (3) the theory of health as a result of the *balance* between four fluids found in a human body, blood, phlegm, yellow and black bile—whilst the disease was the *imbalance* between one or more of these fluids, also referred to as humours; (4) the body's self-healing mechanisms. As such, to understand and treat disease, the Hippocratic writings highlighted the importance of understanding natural processes within a body, that is the physiology of the human body, the significance of observing the body and collecting empirical data for this purpose.

Despite the centuries[2] that break apart the Hippocrates' and Aelius Galenus' eras, their contributions to medicine are deeply intertwined. Galen had a reverence for Hippocratic principles, for which he played an essential role in transmitting Hippocratic medicine to future generations. Moreover, the analogy stated in Plato's *Phaedrus* regarding the whole, which should not be reduced to its parts, is later questioned by Galen, who underlined the importance of understanding a body's constituent parts: "[T]he Hippocratic school tended in some degree to overlook the importance of its constituent parts" [20, p. xii].

The Hippocrates era followed the Asklepios cult influences, making the transition from physical dysfunctions treated by god Asklepios to ones treated by humans known by the title "physician," as it appears in *The Politics of Aristotle* [21] when mentioning Hippocrates "(...) in the same sense of great in which Hippocrates might be called greater, not as a man, but as a *physician*, than someone else who was taller" (Politiká, VII.4, 1326a4). Between the fourth and fifth centuries BC, theories focussed on understanding the mechanisms behind medical conditions, and the methods based on observations were designed for diagnosing and predicting. Galen, in particular, adopted and further developed Hippocratic theories [18, 20]. One of the theories was based on the body's capacity to adjust itself when placed in new conditions by "giving Nature a chance" [18, pp. 1286–7, 20, pp. xi–xii].

Therefore, we can assert that during Hippocrates and continuing with Galen, there was a paradigm change from the "divine paradigm" to the "natural forces paradigm," pivotal in shifting from a blind, divine perspective of explaining the disease to a logical method of examination based on observation. Galen later brought not a change in understanding the disease but a perspective regarding the whole by reducing it to its parts and then considering the whole by adding up the acquired knowledge of the parts.

[2] Hippocrates lived around 460 BC to 370 BC, whilst Galen lived from 129 AD to c. 200 or 216 AD.

5.3 The Second Paradigm Shift: From the "Natural Forces" to the "Reductionist" Paradigm

The foundation laid by Greek philosophy in medicine evolved into the biomedical model [19]. Whilst scientific and objective, this model was less reductionist than its contemporary understanding and set the stage for modern biomedical emphasis on understanding diseases through biological mechanisms, finding universal cures. The biomedical model was further propelled by Descartes in the seventeenth century, who continued to influence the separation of mind and body in medical thinking through philosophical dualism.

The biomedical model (BMM), currently considered traditional, is also a tacit consequence of the Cartesian theory (1642) associated with the Newtonian (1687) mechanical approach [22–26]—as derived from *Philosophiæ Naturalis Principia Mathematica* [27]. Whilst Descartes separated the mind from the body, the Newtonian view applied later in medicine in the Enlightenment era reduced the patient's clinical features to malfunctions of body parts as a machine, where the disease is a mechanical malfunction. The Cartesian and Newtonian underpinnings on which the BMM rests have consistently shaped medicine since the seventeenth century.

Moreover, the emergence of modern, Western scientific medicine, characterised by its mechanistic view of the human body and disease through biomedical precepts, aligns with Weber's broader concept of rationalisation that distinguishes among types of rationality: practical, theoretical, substantive and formal [28]. Because Weber's theory emphasises calculability, predictability and control, it represents the transition towards a more structured, systematic approach by applying scientific knowledge through methodical procedures to improve patient care, diagnosis and treatment. Hewa and Hetherington [28] connect Max Weber's theory of rationalisation to models of medicine by examining the development of the mechanistic biomedical model within the context of rationalisation processes in history. In addition, Weber's influence[3] can be observed in the standardisation of medical protocols and evidence-based practices, such as the development of medical guidelines.

Towards the end of the twentieth century, translational medicine (TM) was introduced to translate scientific discoveries from basic biomedical research into practical application [29]. This approach encompasses the process of translating research evidence into clinical trials. TM aims to bridge the gap between laboratory discovery from biomedicine and clinical implementation, to develop new diagnostics, treatments and preventive strategies to address unmet clinical needs; it builds upon discoveries in biomedicine by transferring scientific evidence to clinical applications [30–32]. Moreover, TM started as a bench-to-bedside, from laboratory to clinical practice, and developed into "a two-way road" bench-to-bedside and bedside-to-bench medicine [31]. Basic research in biomedicine elucidates disease's

[3] That focusses on efficiency and predictability through adherence to universal standards and procedures.

molecular and cellular mechanisms, identifies potential therapeutic targets and informs the development of new interventions. Thus, biomedicine and translational medicine took an integrated approach to advancing medical science and improving patient care. Biomedicine provided the foundational knowledge, and translation medicine facilitated the translation of research discoveries into clinical innovations. In other words, biomedicine generated the foundational knowledge and discoveries that served as the basis for translational research.

Therefore, the shift from "natural forces" to a "reductionist" paradigm, although initiated in the seventeenth and eighteenth centuries by Descartes and Newton, has persisted. Towards the end of the twentieth century, this reductionist paradigm was not only a research model but was also transposed in clinical settings, connecting the bench to bedside medicine and vice versa. The result was visible in further enhancements of medical knowledge.

5.4 The Third Paradigm Shift: From "Reductionist" to "Holistic"?

5.4.1 Initial Stages

In opposition to the reductionist, mechanistic biomedical model (BMM) of research, the biopsychosocial model (BPSM) was first introduced as a solution to the crisis that George Engel asserted to be present in "all medicine" due to "the adherence to a model of disease no longer adequate for the scientific tasks and social responsibilities of either medicine or psychiatry"[4] [33, p. 129].

Engel grounded his biopsychosocial model in several scientific aspects that challenged the reductionist and mechanistic views of the traditional biomedical model. He drew upon Ludwig von Bertalanffy's General Systems Theory (GST), which presents a holistic framework for understanding and analysing complex systems [34]. Therefore, through the GST, it is understood that various systems (biological, mechanical, social, etc.) share common organising principles and can be studied using a unified approach. This theory contrasts with the reductionist methodologies, which analyse systems by breaking them into constituent parts. Instead, to understand the behaviour and properties of a system, GST underlines the importance of looking at the entire system, which means also the interactions between its parts. Under Bertalanffy's theory, Engel grounds his holistic approach to understanding life processes. As such, Engel considers it essential to widen the spectrum of knowledge by putting together all levels of organisation, from molecular to societal, and

[4] What is worth noting here is that in the 1970s, psychiatry was not considered a branch of medical practice specialties but a "discipline based on behavioral science" [33, p. 129]. The discussion over whether psychiatry belonged to medicine started during the 1970s, and later, its principles were reinforced in general medical practice [3, 49, 50].

acknowledging the interconnections and interactions between them. Therefore, he highlights that to facilitate a complete understanding of health and disease, it is important to recognise patterns and principles across these levels and a patient's biological, psychological and social dimensions.

Engel critiques the biomedical model for its emphasis on molecular biology and its failure to account for the complexities of human health, which, he considers, cannot be fully understood through reductionist methods alone. He argues that integrating principles from General Systems Theory into the biopsychosocial approach would develop a more effective framework for medical research and practice through acknowledging the interconnectedness of different levels of the organisation and the role of psychosocial determinants on health and disease. His critique extends to the scientific methodology of the biomedical model, pointing out its limitations in addressing the full spectrum of factors that influence health.

This shift towards a holistic understanding of health for advancing medical science is seen as essential in improving patient care, as biomedicine is. Since Engel advocates for a broader, more integrative view of medicine, he challenges the biomedical paradigm. He considers that his view would reflect human life's and health's complexity. He was, thus, making the case for a fundamental reorientation in how disease and health are conceptualised and addressed within the medical community . Engel argued that effective healthcare must go beyond treating biological dysfunction, including understanding the patient's psychological state and social environment, a strong consideration of the patient's overall well-being and the multifaceted influences on their health. Moreover, it is about therapeutic strategies tailored to each patient to address the biological underpinnings of disease and the psychosocial aspects that can impact patient recovery and quality of life, endorsing a more patient-centred approach to medicine.

Understanding a patient's stress factors and coping mechanisms can be as crucial as identifying the proper medication. Therefore, from Engel's perspective, physicians and healthcare providers should incorporate an awareness regarding all patient dimensions: their mental health, emotional state, family dynamics, cultural background and socioeconomic status. Consequently, fostering a therapeutic relationship between the patient and the healthcare provider would improve patient outcomes, because the patient would comply with treatment plans. In addition, it would make it possible to address potential barriers to recovery that may arise from the patient's psychosocial context.

George Engel's position can be interpreted as transposing bench medicine to bedside medicine by emphasising the integration of scientific findings from the laboratory (bench) to clinical practice (bedside) through a non-reductionist understanding of the patient, an inclusive approach that recognises not only the biological aspects of disease but also the psychological and social factors that influence health outcomes. Overall, Engel's biopsychosocial model calls for including training in psychology, sociology, and communication skills alongside traditional biomedical sciences.

Suppose we put in conjunction with Engel's considerations the new research findings regarding the connection between mind and body, that is personalised medicine and psychoneuroimmunology. In that case, we are looking at an informed shift from an objective disease-centred medicine (biomedical) to one that recognises the subject of medicine, the patient, holistically, with all in favour of patient-centred medicine.

5.4.2 Later Stages

In recent years, the need for integrative and individualised evidence-based medicine that could objectify the interplay amongst biological, psychological and social factors has registered a significant awareness [35, 36] through personalised medicine and psychoneuroimmunoendocrinology.

On the one hand, personalised medicine (PM) recognises the importance of individual variability and considers multiple biological, psychological and social factors developed from the Human Genome Project's applicability to pharmacogenetics [37–39]. Known also as precision or individualised medicine, PM customises medical interventions according to a person's genetic makeup, lifestyle and environmental factors [40]. It offers a more specific application using advanced technologies and data analysis to develop highly targeted and individualised treatments according to a patient's specific molecular and genetic characteristics and medical history [39]. This customisation is made possible by sequencing the individual's genome and adjusting drug dosages based on the likelihood of potential adverse reactions specific to that individual. Subsequently, because of the assets that PM presents, it can also focus on prevention. PM thus acknowledges the significance of individual variability and diverse factors in health and disease, indicating a shift towards a holistic medicine centred on the uniqueness of each patient. In this sense, it can be considered a proper patient-centred approach to healthcare. Its weaknesses are high costs, limited availability, complexity in data analysis, genetic testing, collaboration amongst multiple specialities, complex decision making and data privacy [38].

On the other hand, there is a systematic work offered by an interdisciplinary field that explores the interactions amongst the psychological, nervous, endocrine and immune systems and how these interactions influence health and disease, also known as psychoneuroimmunology or Psycho-Neuro-Endocrine-Immunology (PNEI). Although PNEI is still a relatively new domain, it has a vital role in understanding and explaining the mind-body connection and how this affects health and disease. Research has shown that psychological and social factors can affect the immune system and raise the risk of developing different health problems, including infectious diseases, autoimmune disorders and cancer [3, 4, 41, 42]. Stress hormones, like cortisol, and the dysregulation of immune cell activity are the basis of this interconnection amongst the nervous, endocrine and immune systems [43]. However, the clinical applications of PNEI research are still in the early stages. More research is needed to fully understand the complex interactions between these systems and their effects on health and disease. Although PNEI is still an emerging field, its findings are increasingly used in medicine. For example studies have suggested that stress management techniques, such as mindfulness meditation, may improve immune function and reduce the risk of illness [44, 45].

The biopsychosocial model integrates biological, psychological and social factors to understand health and disease. In contrast, the biomedical model focusses more narrowly on purely biological aspects of disease and treatment. Since PNEI examines how psychological states (like stress and emotions), the nervous system, the endocrine system and the immune system interact and influence each other to affect an individual's overall health, it follows that PNEI has a holistic view regarding a person's physiology. This field acknowledges the complexity of the human condition, emphasising that it cannot be fully understood or treated by looking at biological factors alone—it integrates the mind-body connection with the social environment in which an individual lives. Also, PNEI supports the idea that effective treatment must address the biological mechanisms of disease and the psychological and social contexts that influence the individual's health. PNEI is increasingly recognised as essential for developing more effective medical interventions, promoting well-being, and understanding the multifaceted nature of human health and disease. Psycho-neuro-immuno-endocrinology, thus, operates as a biopsychosocial rather than strictly a biomedical research model.

The complexity of individual differences gives rise to limitations and challenges of PNEI, a lack of standardised methodologies and practical interventions [4]. Continued advancements in technology and methodology could lead to a better understanding of the mind-body connection and its implications for health and disease.

Although it covers other aspects besides the biological characteristics by being customised to a person's personal genetic makeup and internal and external factors that may contribute to the occurrence, development and treatment of a disease, PM is still considered to be rooted in a reductionist approach of health and disease [40] due to its focus at the molecular level. However, we can assert that precision medicine is the most holistic of the biomedical research models and the most reductionist of the biopsychosocial research models, whilst not losing sight of the whole. In contrast, PNEI is the most holistic of the integrative research fields regarding how health and disease are scientifically approached.

5.5 Paradigm Shifts in Medical Practice and Education: Are Bedside Practice and Education Aligned to Bench Medicine?

The BMM-guided approach favours the patient's extraction from their multifaceted personal milieu by bringing their health-disease image into a "one-size-fits-all" frame. What happened was that the patient was no longer a unique individual but rather a statistical figure. Their identity as a person who suffers from an illness was discarded, and only the biological aspects were visible to the biomedical researcher or the biomedical-guided physician. This automatic extraction may be equally seen as an ex vivo setting in contrast with an in vivo setting. The capacity to determine the molecular cause of a disease is a tremendous technological achievement. Once the body is extracted from its context, that is psychological features, the natural and social environment, and its related behaviour, it will shift from an in vivo to an ex vivo investigation. As such, if further advances would not include a person's environmental influences and psychological features, this method of inquiry would lead to disconnection from the body's inner physiological mechanisms and its actual reality in space.

We concluded that modern medical branches that adopt a biopsychosocial view, like personalised medicine and psycho-neuro-endocrine-immunology, see the patient holistically. Regarding PM, derived from the capacity of sequencing the human genome, the researchers agreed upon the importance and the dynamic elements that vary from one person to another, such as "genotype, epigenetic effects, endogenous influences, environmental factors, and microbiome differences" [46, p. 473]. From a distinct perspective but with the same holistic view, PNEI addresses a patient's medical condition through its multidisciplinary approach. Although PM and PNEI have brought a more holistic perspective in understanding health and disease, they are still emerging fields that stumble due to the complexity they encompass, which is related to the lack of standardised methodologies and the financial implications. These aspects limit the fields' spread and contestability, which, in contrast, the traditional biomedical research model lacks.

Reaching a greater understanding of a living organism through social and psychological factors alongside molecular biology and genetics, with applicability in pharmacogenetics, may be considered a paradigm shift in medicine. This shift was possible due to medical technological advancements that, paradoxically, reduced the body even more. In this case, the reduction went even further than what was initially considered "its parts." In the past, these parts were the result of dividing the body into its systems and organs, thus macroscopic. The intermediate step was to identify the molecular components of a cell using the microscope. More recently, the inquiry was pursued on a nuclear level through genomics and molecular biology.

Since the development of fields such as precision medicine and psycho-neuro-endocrine-immunology was possible because of the recent technological advancements in medical research, the reductionist-holistic debate remains far from over. There is no consensus regarding the extent to which each adopts a reductionist or holistic approach. The reason resides in their distinct impact on clinical practice: the biomedical perspective line of defence favours reductionism, whilst the biopsychosocial perspective tends towards holism. However, both fields often employ reductionist methods in studying each system or establishing connections between biological, emotional, and social components, despite their holistic aim of understanding the patient's genetic makeup or mind-body connection.

5.6 Mentality Rather Than a Paradigm Shift

As stated, the biomedical model relies on the theory that biological factors cause diseases and resides in Max Weber's rationalised theory. In contradistinction, the biopsychosocial model relies on the theory that a combination of psychological and social aspects, besides the biological, determines health and illness, based on the General System Theory [28]. As shown, integrating Max Weber's theory of rationalisation in medicine and the distinctions in rationality—practical, theoretical, substantive and formal—into the mechanistic biomedical model showcases how this model exemplifies the move towards a more systematic, evidence-based approach in healthcare. It is considered that through Weber's concepts of formal rationality, medicine is now focussing on the importance of calculability, predictability and control, hence the standardisation of medical protocols and the push towards efficiency and effectiveness in patient care.

In conjunction with the Newtonian mechanical approach, the Cartesian theory influences and favours the patient's depersonalisation through the physician's inertia given by biomedical-oriented educational and professional collective medical knowledge. Moreover, the Cartesian and Newtonian legacy in medicine promotes simplifying physiological processes into mechanical interactions. These propagated perspectives continue to influence medical research and practice because their input to modern medicine has not been disputed by the new advancements made in the past decades. These views embedded in the BMM correlate to the physician's approach to a patient [47, 48]. Therefore, practitioners who adhere to the BMM restrict understanding a patient's physiology to mechanical interactions—the Newtonian perspective of viewing organisms as the sum of their parts. These conceptions, therefore, are deeply ingrained in medical education due to the longstanding and undisputed tradition in medical practice. Consequently, it is challenging to shift away from these concepts, leading some practitioners to favour them over the more recent humanistic approach, which prioritises the patient's perspective. Moreover, the contamination of bedside medicine from lines of inquiry within bench medicine has proven the confusion in the doctor-patient relationship.

However, the interaction between physician and patient occurs on multiple levels. These levels include physical contact during the examination and various forms of communication. All these form the cornerstone of clinical evaluations and medical history collection. Physical interaction is most common due to the inherent nature of physical examinations, followed closely by communication, which encompasses verbal, nonverbal and paraverbal forms. Whilst physical and communicative interactions enrich a clinical exam, a notable knowledge gap exists regarding the cognitive interactions between clinicians and patients. In these interactions, the medical professional seeks to collect essential health information from the patient through dialogue—the patient provides information to receive medical care. In short, the patient plays a passive role in receiving treatment after being provided the information the doctor requested. This dynamic can lead to an automatic behavioural response, where the patient, through disempowerment, enables the clinician to take charge of the treatment. We are thus talking about a dynamic that disrupts the reciprocal flow of information, which leads to a power imbalance and an asymmetric relationship. Despite a trend toward adopting a more self-empowering approach, the cognitive dimension of their interaction with clinicians remains insufficiently examined.

Due to easy access to information, the modern patient can access a heavy informational load, which can clutter the doctor-patient dialogue because the physician has to clarify the patient's image of their disease, including treatment options and possible outcomes. On the other hand, there is the legitimate, well-informed patient, the physician-as-patient, who needs no extra clarification, in which case, the physician's goal consists of guiding the patient to make the right decision concerning their medical condition—an in-depth analysis is provided in Chaps. 6 and 7.

Considering these distinct categories of patient information processing, we can identify various approaches to illness from the patient's perspective. First, there is the patient who fully entrusts the physician with the authority to decide how to address the illness. Second, there is the patient who does not critically evaluate the credibility or source of the information they receive. Finally, the educated patient knows where to seek reliable information (e.g. researching cases related to their diagnosis) and does so with discernment. This patient uses the data to better understand the physician's recommended course of action without undermining the patient-doctor relationship or overstepping the trust in the physician's expertise.

Mentality shift relies on the idea that meaningful advancements in patient outcomes depend less on changing theoretical medical paradigms and more on how practitioners approach their work and relationships with patients. Instead of strictly following rigid, theoretically established models (such as those depicted from the biomedical or biopsychosocial models), a mentality shift would mean a mindset focussed on adaptability, empathy and patient-centred care, changing positions from the outer world to the inner world through cognitive and metacognitive processing.

Within this work frame, practitioners would feel free and encouraged to reflect on their thought processes, biases and interactions with patients. By doing so, they can move beyond rigid, model-based practices and respond more effectively to individual patients' unique needs and contexts whilst also being in tune with their own cognitive and emotional processes. Such a mindset would, therefore, value the integration of scientific rigour with compassionate, holistic care, recognising that patient outcomes improve when care is tailored to them and not just the disease. In addition, healthcare providers would not feel that they need to be stuck in a particular frame when addressing patients' needs.

Empathy allows practitioners to connect with patients on a human level, fostering trust and open communication, which are foundational for effective care. Adaptability enables clinicians to respond dynamically to each patient's unique circumstances rather than rigidly applying general protocols that may not suit individual needs. Comprehensive care recognises patients as whole individuals, not merely as cases defined by symptoms or diagnoses.

For modern medicine to realise its full potential, it is essential to shift from rigid traditional models to a mentality that prioritises compassion, empathy, adaptability and comprehensive patient care. By embracing a mentality shift, healthcare providers may develop, in time, a more flexible, patient-centred approach by becoming aware of a person's experience of illness, disease and suffering.

Ultimately, this mentality shift may bridge the gap between scientific knowledge and compassionate care, ensuring that medicine is innovative and deeply attuned to the humanity of those it serves.

References

1. Scheffler RW, Strasser BJ (2015) Biomedical sciences, history and sociology of. In: International encyclopedia of the social & behavioral sciences, 2nd edn. Elsevier, Orlando. https://doi.org/10.1016/B978-0-08-097086-8.85045-X
2. Kuhn TS (1970) The structure of scientific revolutions, 2nd edn. The University of Chicago Press, Enlarged
3. Bottaccioli F, Bottaccioli AG (2017) Psycho-neuro-endocrino-immunology paradigm and cardiovascular diseases. In: Fioranelli M (ed) Integrative cardiology. Springer, Cham, pp 139–151
4. Bitzer-Quintero OK, Ortiz GG, Jaramillo-Bueno S, Ramos-González EJ, Márquez-Rosales MG, Delgado-Lara DLC, Torres-Sánchez ED, Tejeda-Martínez AR, Ramirez-Jirano J (2022) Psycho-neuro-endocrine-immunology: a role for melatonin in this new paradigm. Molecules. https://doi.org/10.3390/MOLECULES27154888
5. Nundy S, Oswald J (2014) Relationship-centered care: a new paradigm for population health management. Healthcare 2:216–219
6. Bennett Johnson S (2012) Medicine's paradigm shift: an opportunity for psychology. APA 43:5
7. Shulman L (2014) A shifting paradigm—medical to interactional model: a personal history. Adv Soc Work 15:207–229
8. Saad M, de Medeiros R, Mosini AC (2017) Are we ready for a true biopsychosocial–spiritual model? The many meanings of "Spiritual". Medicines 4:79
9. Patel VL, Kaufman DR, Arocha JF (2002) Emerging paradigms of cognition in medical decision-making. J Biomed Inform 35:52–75
10. James CA, Wheelock KM, Woolliscroft JO (2021) Machine learning: the next paradigm shift in medical education. Acad Med 96(7):954–957
11. Brauer S, Kettunen J, Levy A, Merenmies J, Kulmala P (2023) The educational paradigm shift—a phenomenographic study of medical teachers' experiences of practices. BMC Med Educ 23:1–10
12. Naithani N, Vasudevan B (2021) Paradigm shift in medical education: the future beckons. Med J Armed Forces India 77:S1
13. Curnow T (2012) The cult of Asclepius: its origins and early development. Bull John Rylands Univ Libr Manchester 89:67–83
14. Doolittle BR (2021) The philosopher-priest-scientist and the new age of medicine. Am J Med 134:425–427
15. Barnard D (1985) The physician as priest, revisited. J Relig Health 24:272–286
16. Edelstein EJ, Edelstein L (1945) Asclepius: a collection and interpretation of the testimonies. https://doi.org/10.2307/4342353
17. Craik EM (2015) The 'Hippocratic' corpus. Routledge
18. Hippocrates (2015) The complete works of Hippocrates. Delphi Classics
19. Tamm ME (1993) Models of health and disease. Br J Med Psychol 66:213–228
20. Galen (1916) On the natural faculties. Harvard University Press, Cambridge, MA

21. Jowett B (1885) The politics of Aristotle. Oxford University Press
22. Bottaccioli F (2014) La fine della grande illusione del riduzionismo in biologia e in medicina. Epistemologia 37:5–21
23. Spencer D (2017) Narrative medicine. In: Solomon M, Simon JR, Kincaid H (eds) The Routledge companion to philosophy of medicine. Routledge, New York, pp 372–382
24. O'Leary D (2021) Medicine's metaphysical morass: how confusion about dualism threatens public health. Synthese 199:1977–2005
25. Gold J (1985) Cartesian dualism and the current crisis in medicine — a plea for a philosophical approach: discussion paper. J R Soc Med 78:663–666
26. Duncan G (2000) Mind-body dualism and the biopsychosocial model of pain: what did Descartes really say? J Med Philos 25:485–513
27. Newton I (1846) The mathematical principles of natural philosophy (1687). Daniel Adee, New York
28. Hewa S, Hetherington RW (1995) Specialists without spirit: limitations of the mechanistic biomedical model. Theor Med 16:129–139
29. Geraghty J (1996) Adenomatous polyposis coli and translational medicine. Lancet 348:422
30. Monteiro S, Sherbino J, Sibbald M, Norman G (2020) Critical thinking, biases and dual processing: the enduring myth of generalisable skills. Med Educ 54:66–73
31. Keramaris NC, Kanakaris NK, Tzioupis C, Kontakis G, Giannoudis PV (2008) Translational research: from benchside to bedside. Injury 39:643–650
32. Marincola FM (2003) Translational medicine : a two-way road. J Transl Med 2:1–2
33. Engel GL (1977) The need for a new medical model: a challenge for biomedicine. Science 196:129–136
34. von Bertalanffy L (1968) General system theory: foundations, development, applications. George Braziller, New York
35. Stewart M, Belle Brown J, Weston W, Mcwhinney IR, Mcwilliam CL, Freeman TR (2014) Patient-centered medicine transforming the clinical method. Radcliffe Publishing
36. Gartner JB, Abasse KS, Bergeron F, Landa P, Lemaire C, Côté A (2022) Definition and conceptualization of the patient-centered care pathway, a proposed integrative framework for consensus: a concept analysis and systematic review. BMC Health Serv Res 22:1–24
37. Collins FS, Fink L (1995) The human genome project. Alcohol Health Res World 19:190–195
38. Greenhalgh T (2005) The human genome project. J R Soc Med 98:545
39. Gibbs RA (2020) The human genome project changed everything. Nat Rev Genet 21:575–576
40. Delpierre C, Lefèvre T (2023) Precision and personalized medicine: what their current definition says and silences about the model of health they promote. Implication for the development of personalized health. Front Sociol 8:1–5
41. Dinan TG, Cryan JF (2017) Microbes immunity and behavior: psychoneuroimmunology meets the microbiome. Neuropsychopharmacology 42:178–192
42. Irwin MR (2008) Human psychoneuroimmunology: 20 years of discovery. Brain Behav Immun 22:129–139
43. Daruna JH (2012) Introduction to psychoneuroimmunology, 2nd edn. Elsevier
44. Bottaccioli AG, Bottaccioli F, Carosella A, Cofini V, Muzi P, Bologna M (2020) Psychoneuroendocrinoimmunology-based meditation (PNEIMED) training reduces salivary cortisol under basal and stressful conditions in healthy university students: results of a randomized controlled study. EXPLORE 16:189–198
45. Demori I, Grasselli E (2023) The role of the stress response in metabolic dysfunction-associated fatty liver disease: a psychoneuroendocrineimmunology-based perspective. Nutrients 15(3):795
46. Nebert DW, Zhang G (2019) Pharmacogenomics. In: Emery and Rimoin's principles and practice of medical genetics and genomics: foundations. Academic, pp 445–486
47. Tauber AI (2017) Medical humanism. Part 1: philosophical and historical underpinnings. In: Marcum JA (ed) The Bloomsbury companion to contemporary philosophy of medicine. Bloomsbury Academic, London, pp 161–182

48. Fialová L (2017) Medical humanism. Part 2: Inspirations of the twentieth century. In: Marcum JA (ed) The Bloomsbury companion to contemporary philosophy of medicine. Bloomsbury Academic, London, pp 183–204
49. Marcum JA (2008) An introductory philosophy of medicine: humanizing modern medicine. Philos Med. https://doi.org/10.1007/978-1-4020-6797-6
50. Anjum RL, Copeland S, Rocca E (2020) Rethinking causality, complexity and evidence for the unique patient. Springer. https://doi.org/10.1007/978-3-030-41239-5

Part II
On the Doctor's and Patient's Extended Minds

Chapter 6
Extended Mind Theory and the Doctor-Patient Relationship

6.1 Introduction

The Extended Mind Theory (EMT), as described originally by Clark and Chalmers [1], is grounded on the idea that cognition does not rely only on the brain but also on the agent's body and its outer environment. They propose "an active externalism, based on the active role of the environment in driving cognitive processes" [1, p. 7]. By active externalism, they claim that a person relates to "an external entity in a two-way interaction, creating a coupled system that can be seen as a cognitive system in its own right" [1, p. 8]. Consequently, they argue that the elements of this coupled system are in a causal relationship that influences behaviour as much as cognition does. Moreover, they endorse that if it were to remove parts of this system, behavioural competence would decline to a similar extent as it would if parts of the brain were damaged or removed.

Clark and Chalmers propose the "Inga-Otto" thought experiment, arguing that "*beliefs* can be constituted partly by features of the environment when those features play the right sort of role in driving cognitive processes" [1, p. 12]. In short, Inga and Otto are hypothetical characters. Otto has Alzheimer's disease; therefore, he has problems recalling information, whereas Inga is cognitively healthy. To remember how they can reach address B, Inga uses her brain (brain resourced), whereas Otto must write down the steps (paper resourced) that help him get from A to B by following them precisely. In other words, "the notebook plays for Otto the same role that memory plays for Inga" [2, p. 32]. They consider Otto's information retrieved from his notebook as "an ordinary non-occurrent belief" [1, p. 13], concluding that "the information lies beyond the skin" in his notebook [ibid.].

Richard Menary's [3] and Lawrence Shapiro's [4] collection on different perspectives and criticism related to extended mind theory and embodied cognition theory are bringing forward major traits from Clark and Chalmers' work that several opponents of the EMT have criticised. Menary considers that the only

G.-P. Florea, *Metacognition and Medical Humanities in Medical Education*, New Paradigms in Healthcare, https://doi.org/10.1007/978-3-032-01070-4_6

difference between Otto's way (by following the indications as written in his notebook previously) and Inga's way (by using her biological mind as a resource, her brain) of getting to address B is "the location of the information" [3, p. 9], the notebook in Otto's case and the biological brain in Inga's case. Therefore, Otto's mind is extended outside the body, on the notebook, "into the world," and "it just happens that this information lies beyond the skin" [1].

Significant criticisms are related to the active externalism, coupling-constitution argument, extended beliefs, the parity principle and the derived and underived content [3, pp. 1–25], as they seem to be presented in Clark and Chalmers' essay. Based on their view on what they call "Otto two-step" [5, p. 46], Otto's cognitive processes are based on a chronologically grounded series of beliefs that to reach point B, he must look into the notebook, belief number one, and then following the instructions that he previously wrote in his notebook, he will follow belief number two, or "the (new) belief about the actual street address" [3, p. 10]. Menary claims Otto and Inga's memories cannot be "on a par." His objections fall into two categories, one of criticism and another of constructive discussion, which tackles new perspectives that can develop from EM.

Also, in Shapiro's [4] collection, Aizawa presents several criticisms of Clark and Chalmers' coupling-system concept, accepting it as fallacious. He rephrases the entire argument as a mechanism where process *X* causally influences a cognitive process *Y*, assuming further that the whole *X*-*Y* process is a cognitively coupled system. To strengthen the fallacy, Aizawa places the entire argument in a different context: *X* being "the process of evaporative cooling found in a typical home air conditioning" and *Y* a process of "deformation in the shape of a bimetallic strip in a thermostat in one room of the house" [6, p. 35]. Even though the *X* process is in a causal relation to the *Y* process, he asserts that "this causal linkage between *X* and *Y* does not make the entire *X*-*Y* process a process of shape deformation"; therefore, "it does not make the whole *X*-*Y* process a matter of evaporative cooling system" [ibid.]. I consider Aizawa's criticism of the coupling system a weak argument. The effects of mechanical processes cannot be on par with the mental process. The physical and functional key element in Otto's coupling system is his brain, a dynamic organ that receives various inputs from the outer environment. The argument that a mechanical component (the *X* process) is in a causal relation with another mechanical element (the *Y* process), resulting in a shape deformation, cannot be applied in a more complex process—the human mind and its linkage with the external environment with effect on a person's behaviour.

Despite Aizawa's criticism regarding debating the coupling-constitution system, the most argued feature of Clark and Chalmers' work, he stresses its relevancy as "a provocation to further investigation" [6, p. 37]. According to Aizawa, "cognition extends" if and only if "there is the right kind of causal connection between brainy cognitive processes and bodily and environmental processes" [6, p. 35], making possible the extension of cognition. Consequently, he considers the need for a set of additional conditions to make this coupling relation "to suffice to establish constitutive relations."

> It should lead us to ask how to refine the mistaken, simplistic account into a correct, sophisticated account. There are, however, two challenges lurking here. First of all, if we propose that additional conditions, C1, … , Cn, are needed in order for coupling relations to suffice to establish constitutive relations, then we must bear the burden of determining and theoretically validating those additional conditions C1, … , Cn. [6, p. 36]

Following this line of judgement, I describe below the medical encounter between the patient and the physician as having the properties of an environment where one's cognition extends to the other's sensorimotor system under the *right* conditions of this precise setting. There is a counterargument that may reject the "coupling-constitution fallacious" [6, p. 35]. If we consider the cognitive coupled system created between the physician's and the patient's mental processes as a result of their interaction as the underlying mental processes that occur in a placebo response, to propose additional conditions "for the coupling relations to suffice to establish constitutive relations" [ibid.], one should first outline the environment they are referring to and then determine the possibility of a cognitive coupled system to unfold.

6.2 The Coupling System Argument in Medical Practice

Starting from the central claim of this section—the patient and the physician constitute a cognitive system, the patient-physician relationship as a coupling system—let us consider Aizawa's previously presented logical thread in an equation form as it follows:

Let us assume that *X* represents any "process" happening in the environment, and *Y* denotes a "cognitive process."

If

$$X \overset{\text{Causal influence}}{\rightarrow} Y,$$

Then,

$$X + Y = \text{a}(\text{coupled}) \text{ cognitive process}$$

Consequently, if a person's cognitive process (*X*), which results in an action or behaviour, considered *the* environment, has a causal influence on another agent's cognitive process (*Y*), coupled together, the agent's action as a result of their cognitive process and the other agent's cognitive process become a coupled cognitive system.

When talking about the physician-patient interaction, the cognitive system is a structure based on the following two elements:

(1) The process X = physician's action like the physical examination or dialogue with the patient, thus the environment that the patient perceives as such, and

(2) the cognitive process Y = the patient's cognitive process/mind within the medical environment, during the clinical examination or dialogue, when the therapeutic "ritual" is being performed.

What follows is:

<< the patient's cognitive process within the medical environment> > is in a causality rapport with <<physician's action upon the patient through physical examination or dialogue>>

Placing these two elements into the given equation, the latter changes as follows:

<< physician's action > > = *PhA* (considered to be the environment as perceived by the patient)
and << the patient's cognitive process/mind >> = *PM*,

If

$$PhA \overset{\text{Causal influence}}{\rightarrow} PM,$$

Then,
The short logical sequence is:

$$\text{If } PhA \overset{\text{Causal influence}}{\rightarrow} PM, \text{ then } PhA + PM = \text{coupled system}$$

=> physician's action and patient's cognitive process/mind constitute a coupled cognitive system.

Extensively,

PhA+PM = cognitive system => the environment, as it is perceived by the patient, created by the physician's action, constitutes a coupled cognitive system.

According to this logical mapping, a physician's actions causal influence a patient's mind/cognitive process. Equally, a patient's action can influence a physician's mind/cognitive process. Consequently, together, they form a coupled cognitive system, establishing a two-way one. As the notebook plays an essential role for Otto in getting to address B by following his notebook as an extension of his mind, a physician's medical and humane abilities can have a pivotal role in helping patients follow the steps that could take them to point B, namely, the best outcome in their disease or illness.

So far, I have deduced that the coupled system argument is possible when both agents share the same property, *il cogito*. The assertion that the coupled system argument is fallacious does not apply to complex mental processes between two individuals. A physician's cognition could function as a patient's extension of their mind and strongly affect the latter's disease outcome. After transposing the coupled system argument on the patient-physician relationship stance, I further prove the extended mind theory in clinical practice through the placebo effect. Ab initio, it is necessary to point out different categories of patients and distinguish between types of mental or cognitive bonding that can be created between the physician and the patient in other stands.

6.3 Typologies of Patients According to Their Cognitive Determination

The differences between levels of mental awareness or consciousness among patients must be analysed, since some have limited or impaired cognitive capacity, physiologically or pathologically, and others, like physicians-as-patients, are "exceedingly" aware due to their professional background. This can cloud the physician-as-patient reasoning and perhaps even the doctor's capacity to get to what can be called "informed clinical decision-making."

No matter the disease or illness, mentally reliable patients possess the basic cognitive apparatus that helps them understand their health status and its implications. Moreover, this category of patients can manifest their willpower on what type of treatment suits them best based on the information they receive from the physician (shared decision-making process). According to Benedetti, "the clinician must consider a symptom not so much as a single and isolated entity, but rather within the psychological and social context of the patient" [7, p. 53]. In this line of thought, one's physiological dysfunction manifestation should be investigated within the "holistic individuality" frame, which implies all mental, psychological, social and biological dimensions. Grouping all patients seen by a healthcare provider under the Gaussian bell-shaped curve,[1] without acknowledging that some may fall at the extremes of this statistical distribution, implies treating medicine as a one-size-fits-all practice. Suppose a physician views all patients as fitting within the Gaussian bell-shaped curve without recognising that some may fall at the extremes of this statistical distribution. In that case, it suggests an approach to medicine that treats it as a one-size-fits-all practice.

Firstly, if we consider conscious patients without mental pathology, we must ponder their epistemological content. If the patient does not have a medical background, they could not possibly have the same medical-oriented thinking as a person from the medical guild has. If they are a medical professional, we are talking about a particular case, the doctor-as-a-patient. A medical-knowledgeable patient's cognitive processes differ quantitatively and qualitatively from those in a non-medical person's mind. I use the "lay patient" syntagm to reference the category of patients with a minimum or no medical background. Therefore, due to the reasoning complexity, the difference in mental processing between a lay patient and a

[1] In this case, a standardisation which offers a symmetrical distribution being interpreted as the probability of a patient to have the same symptoms and signs as the majority of patients with the same disease.

physician-as-a-patient requires a distinct approach. Secondly, if discussing unconscious patients or mentally ill patients, the capability of using their minds in rapport with the physiological dysfunction (s) changes the entire approach. When the patient is unconscious, they cannot have a mental judgement, whereas if they are in an altered mental state, a rational process cannot be performed. Therefore, the categories that one can distinguish from are (1) mentally healthy or cognitively reliable patients (lay patients and physicians-as-patients) and (2) mentally non-reliable patients (unconscious patients and psychiatric patients).

The situations presented above show the variety of patients who depend on different mental capacities to understand their physiological dysfunction and the possibilities of being part of the shared decision-making process. Why are these differences so significant? Modern medicine tends towards diminishing paternalism and integrating the patient in the medical decision process. If so, the cognitive coupled system a physician forms with a mentally healthy patient would be altered compared to the mentally absent (unconscious) or mentally ill patient (psychiatric patient). In such cases, family members become the extension of the patient's mind, indirectly making the physician-patient cognitive coupling system form differently. The unconscious or mentally ill patient will be bypassed, and the relation determining the coupled system will have a dissimilar ending point from a cognitive perspective. In this case, the interaction with the patient is no longer bidirectional; it is transformed into a tertiary person-oriented type of relation. Therefore, it changes from a patient-physician relationship to a "third party-physician" relationship, not making it any less. It just moves the centre of cognitive processing to a different person with the effect still on the patient's outcome due to the decisions this third party has to make when the sufferer is in a critical medical stage, for example the decision a person has to make in the patient's name faced with a life and death situation.

Furthermore, in the analogy regarding Clark and Chalmers' coupling system argument and the physician-patient relationship, the distinction between the differences mentioned earlier in mental processes during a medical examination is worth noting. These differences are given, as considered above, by various patients' or third parties' levels of understanding or beliefs.

6.4 Inga-Otto and the Doctor-Patient Thought Experiments

As previously proven, the physician must apply the knowledge stored within their mind. They retrieve theoretical, implicit and explicit knowledge based on experience amassed in their biological mind. Judging from the Inga-Otto case, the physician has mainly Inga's type of resources, the biological mind (brain). Even if, at times, the doctor may need to access biomedical paper resources (scientific papers) when experiencing difficulties remembering hard information, we cannot assert that the physician uses paper resources as Otto does. Suppose Otto needs to recall simple actions like getting from A to B, following step-by-step written indications. In that case, the physician must make complex memory retrievals from a vast quantity of scientific (knowledge-based) and empirical (experience-based) information. As mentioned above, the doctor is the brain-resourced person from the patient-physician couple. Therefore, the physician plays Inga's role in this mental experiment. Patient resources require several aspects that need to be analysed. Even so, we can intuitively assert that the patient can play Otto's role just by thinking he is *the* most dependent person on the outer environment, be it paper or other's memory.

In Otto's case, the notebook can be considered passive input because once written in the notebook, the information does not change. In contrast, the information inside the patient's mind can vary depending on the nature of their feelings, negative or positive [8]. When under emotional stress, one is prone to have one's attention narrowed, and when being in a positive emotional charge, one has one's attention broadened [9, 10]. Therefore, a more complex topic needs to be analysed: how a patient's perception changes when listening to information from the physician, depending on the perspective of the negative or positive diagnosis.

As previously proven, the doctor is part of the coupling cognitive system and the patient within the medical environment. Moreover, different types of mental attributes were designated to various categories of patients. Based on the resources both actors of the thought experiment used in this specific medical circumstance, it implies that the physician is Inga's homolog, and the patient is Otto's counterpart. Physician unequivocally uses brainy resources when performing their profession. Even so, at times, they could use papery resources to find the right solutions due to the complexity of epistemic knowledge they should consider and not because of having problems in brain resources retrieval of information. However, a particular category of patients may be an exception to the general rule; the coupling cognitive system in patient-physician encounters is more rigid in physician-as-a-patient situations. In the category of mentally reliable patients, we may find the following division: (1) the lay patient who has a functional mental apparatus but does not possess medical knowledge, and (2) the physician-as-patient, the patient belonging to the medical guild, with an epistemic background in medicine. Nevertheless, what these two categories have in common is their neural network activated due to the sickness-suppressing-motivated behaviour [7] as presented above.

6.4.1 *Case 1: Physician-Lay Patient Interaction vs. Inga-Otto Mental Experiment*

As stated previously, lay patients must rely on the physician's knowledge to receive the correct diagnosis and adequate treatment. If Otto is paper-resourced, the lay patient is "physician-resourced". As Otto relies on the information from his notebook, so does the patient depend on the physician's memory for retrieving the correct information to reach the best health status outcome. This conclusion follows from the dependent relationship between Otto and his notebook and the dependent relationship between the patient and the physician. At the same time, the physician is following Inga's brain-based resource because the former does not rely on other external resources but mainly on their memory. If we follow this line of judgement, the physician is the cognitive extension for the lay patient due to the mental internal processes that they (the physician), as a specialist, must deliver the proper diagnosis and treatment.

The knowledge transfer framework between the physician and the patient is captured in the following loop, Diagram 6.1. Physician—lay patient knowledge framework:

Step 1—The signs and symptoms coming from the lay patient (from direct and indirect communication) are integrated and processed further by the physician's mind.

Step 2—The information the physician considers communicating to the lay patient to help them achieve the desired outcome following the right therapeutic strategy (lifestyle changes, medications, etc.).

The lay patient depends on the physician's knowledge and even on their authority, and the physician relies on their scientific (knowledge-based) and implicit (experience-based) information, which they retrieve from their memory. When the patient's objective is to reach a better health status, the data coming from the physician equals the information that Otto needs to reach point B by retrieving them from the notebook. Nevertheless, it is worth noting an important distinction: the patient relies only on the information they receive from the physician—as they are given to them by the free will of the physician or at their request—and also, the former later recalls the information based on the dialogue had with the doctor. On the other hand, physicians have a different attitude when sick, based on the vast understanding of what a physiological dysfunction could determine, pathology's consequences and complications. Therefore, the information that the patient remembers depends on the emotional charge of the discussion with the physician.

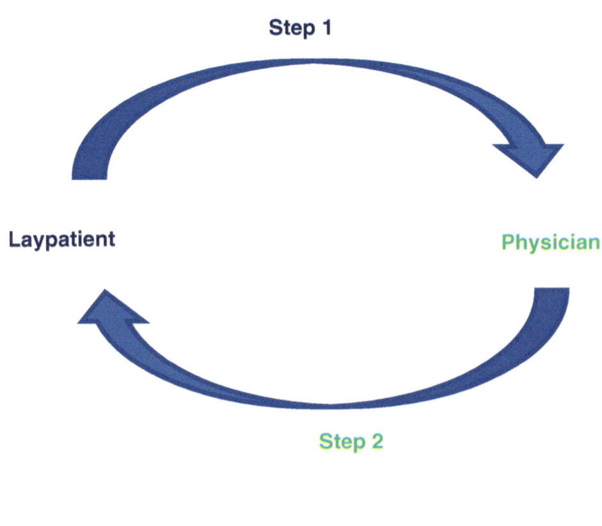

Diagram 6.1 Physician—lay patient knowledge framework

Consider the patient being Otto (O_p) and the patient's memory being Otto's notebook (N_p). If O_p registers within the N_p the information he hears or sees during the meeting with his physician, he can access and retrieve this information at any given time. The information as he records in his N_p at that precise moment will be "read" by O_p with the exact connotation. Even outside the physician's office, he will have access to this information and follow the directions to reach point B, the physiological disfunction's outcome, according to the steps he wrote in his N_p under the physician's guidance. Therefore, if accepting the argument that the patient is in a coupling cognitive system with the physician, the O_p task to reach point B will be dependent on how (1) O_p recorded the directions given by the physician but also on (2) the way he interpreted the details received from the physician. Therefore, based on Clark and Chalmers' view that "*beliefs* can be constituted partly by features of the environment, when those features play the right sort of role in driving cognitive processes" [1, p. 12], the information stored within the N_p can be considered O_p's beliefs.

Furthermore, according to Menary's objection, O_p's cognitive processes are based on a chronologically grounded series of beliefs that to reach point B, he must look into the N_p, belief number one, and then follow the instructions that he previously recorded on his N_p he will have belief number two, or the *new* belief about the actual "destination," better health status in this case. Therefore, I agree with Menary's objection that Otto and Inga's memories cannot be "on a par," as much as O_p's memory cannot be on par with the physician's memory related to how he passed on the medical information. Nevertheless, this account does not make the demonstration less plausible, but it highlights the importance of how the doctor breaks the bad news and medical information. The latter's ability to deliver bad news could alter, or not, how a patient gets to point B, which is the supreme goal that any physician should have, namely, the best outcome for a patient's physiological dysfunction.

6.4.2 *Case 2: Physician—"Physician-as-a-Patient" Versus Inga-Otto Mental Experiment*

Added to what lay patients experience during their illness, physicians-as-patients have more complex behaviour. Within medical literature, it is known that medical professionals behave differently than laypeople do [11–14].

> When a doctor gets sick, his status changes. No longer is his role defined as deriving from *doctus*, i.e., learned, but as from *patients*, the present participle of the deponent verb, *patior*, i.e., to suffer, with all the passive acceptance of pain the verb implies. From *passus*, the past participle, we get the word *passion*, with its wide gamut of emotional allusions, ranging from animal lust to the sufferings of martyrs. It is the connotation, not the denotation, of the word that defines the change of status. [12, p. vii]

In their medical narrative book, Mandell and Spiro (1988) point out what physicians experience when becoming patients [12]. After presenting different medical conditions of 50 cases of physicians-as-patients, they extract essential concerns that these "doctor-patients"[2] have, shaping their general psychological profile based on the common features they manifest during their illness. Therefore, "doctors are often difficult patients" [12, p. 432] and being the physician of a doctor as a patient is a challenging task. There is an unwritten law that most medical students confirm being hypochondriacal during medical school. As Mandell and Spiro underline, after a maniacal period, physicians change perspectives, and "most physicians learn to believe themselves invulnerable" [ibid.]. They also highlight the denial attitude that may be a "trained response of medical school, and the distance of our colleagues" [12, p. 451]. Their analogy between the white coat, which symbolises power, and the hospital gown, which may give rise to humility, is a strong metaphor for the shift between the powerful physician and the weak and vulnerable position the patient, no matter their profession, takes when ill. If the lay patient lives with the idea that they are not immortal, physicians experience it only when they are no longer on "God's throne" once descending from it and becoming the sufferer. From this instance, one can observe the physician's downgrading from the empowered to the powerless.

For a physician, now a patient, transitioning from a powerful, authoritarian professional to a mortal one is mostly impossible. They are going through depersonalisation by embracing the hospital's uniform and needing to obey the system's rules [14, 15]. From being in control of patients' conditions all their careers, they must now give away this position and let other professionals be in charge of their diagnosis and treatment. They lose the alleged control over the physiological dysfunction and are challenged to develop control over the person, the self. Because this process of giving away the power and taking the place of the compliant and non-judgemental patient is a difficult task, physicians as patients often do not receive the correct diagnosis.

> The doctor-patient usually thinks he knows the diagnosis, even if it is the wrong one. Ordinary patients have confidence in their physician's skill, but the medical training of physician-patients gets in their way. They never really accept, never really are given, the chance to be just a patient. Moreover, for the doctor's doctor there is always a sense of fraternity, an immediate merger of identities with physicians. [12, p. 434]

This diagnostic error is due to the physician-as-patient's description of symptoms and their often misleading interpretation. Added to this is the phenomenon of the physician who treats the doctor, who reaches a state of sympathy (and not empathy or compassion) that determines the physician's physician does not have a right, objective view about the knowledgeable patient's health status.

> Immediately the sick physician becomes us. We view his illness as our illness, we merge-as the psychoanalyst might put it-in a final confrontation with our own illness. Our past, our

[2] Using this syntagm, "doctor-patient" is to denote the role of the physician (doctor) as patient and not the doctor-patient relationship.

> present, and our future confront us in the body of the sick physician. It is such a reversal of the natural order of things. Even reading about a doctor's travails with disease is different for a doctor from reading about what another patient might have to say, for we know the doctor understands what is going on better than the layman. [12, p. 435]

Also, physicians-as-patients might hide critical information to avoid making themselves vulnerable in front of their colleagues (underdiagnosis) or because of their hypochondriacal reactions (overdiagnosis). Consequently, this fact determines the wrong treatment.

> It felt appropriate and safe when I discussed my chest growth from a clinical point of view. The familiar role kept my fear at bay and allowed me some comfort in spite of the life-shattering diagnoses we invariably discussed. As long as I could play doctor to my disease, I learned I could at least partially protect myself from the anxiety and feelings of helplessness that accompanied my new status. [14, p. 91]

As the physician's stories reveal, they "try hard to be 'good'," obedient and "docile" patients. They consider that a good patient, even though suffering, should not complain. Sometimes, "they rebel, cry out, leave the hospital early, or ask for second or third opinions" [12, p. 434]. Nevertheless, the majority remains silent, although they know enough to be concerned about.

> Try as we may to be "good," doctors are sometimes "bad" patients because we know the worst. The general surgeon with regional enteritis is more depressed than most because he has seen only the extremes of perforation, obstruction, and abscess. [ibid.]

Nevertheless, from being ill and having the insight of a knowledgeable patient, they have revelations on how important it is to listen to the clues that patients offer when complaining about specific symptoms.

> ... when they fall sick, from the new perspective of patient, most doctors are delighted to discover new diagnostic clues in their own symptoms. They learn how a patient feels and a doctor reacts. [ibid.]

They also underline the difference between the physician who experienced the patient's vulnerability from their own experience and the medical student who had been a patient before their medical school admission.

> The youngster who has been chronically ill brings different conceptions with him to medical school. Some of the patients with inflammatory bowel disease in this volume keep statistics, as if for them the good life was not baseball but enemas. [ibid.]

Furthermore, this information shows us how empathy can be learned through experience capacity or if there is any possibility for empathy to be an already-born ability.

> After so many years of teaching others how to take care of patients, he had no confidence that anyone can know the heart and soul of another. Empathy for him was a metaphor, not a reality. [ibid.]

The purpose of introducing the above excerpts from Mandell and Spiro's book from the 50 physicians' stories regarding their own experiences as patients is to show how their drama differs from that of a lay patient whose fear is mainly based on the unknown, whilst the physician-as-patients main fear is of the most critical unknown.

This collection gathers experienced doctors who suffered from an illness sometime in adulthood. The underlying message that can be extracted from all stories relates to how those experiences change their perception of disease from a subjective position. On the other hand, the understanding of having experienced an illness they or somebody they care for earlier in their lives can represent a strong motivation for choosing medicine to be their profession. This subjective knowledge about suffering and disease acquired through the experience as a patient or as the relative of a suffering person may contribute to the foundation of what James Marcum called the dualistic/holistic metaphysical position worldview of medicine, belonging to the humanistic model he framed it [16, pp. 17–31].

As Myers and Gabbard asserted, perfectionism, self-recrimination, narcissism, arrogance and histrionic characteristics are frequent among medical school students "[s]hy and avoidant of social relatedness (…) arrogant and narcissistic as a way of dealing with their insecurity (…), histrionic and attention seeking (…), antisocial features that lead to corrupt practices later in their careers" [11, p. 4]. The common traits for all physicians and undergraduate students are perfectionism and conscientiousness. These are essential features that make them succeed in this profession.

> (…) perfectionistic behaviors may be desired by patients and rewarded within the field while being personally expensive. (…) perfectionism leads to thorough and comprehensive diagnostic efforts, the systemic ordering of laboratory tests to rule out the most exotic disorders, and detailed planning that takes advantage of the latest innovations in treatment. [ibid.]

According to Myers and Gabbard's description, the causes for possessing a high sense of perfectionism rely on childhood factors (temperament, attachment style), their parents when young (parenting style, personality) and environmental pressures from peers, culture and teachers. Nevertheless, perfectionism is a blade with two edges. It helps in avoiding diagnostic errors by thinking critically. Still, at the same time, perfectionism triggers depression, burnout, suicide and anxiety [11, 17, 18] due to the personal internal pressure under which physicians exert the profession. Future research is needed to see how the propensity for conscious metacognitive processes depends on personality types.

"Medical culture" is another element that Myers and Gabbard analyse to understand the behaviour determinants for physicians-as-patients better. In short, how undergraduate students understand a doctor's daily life, as they see it during their schooling, is essential to their future behavioural development as physicians. Due to how previous generations evolved, physicians construed themselves within the frames of self-sacrifice measured by the hours spent in the clinic. This element is passed on to future generations by imitating the same behaviour. Based on the previously observed standard features among people who submit to medical schools, perfectionism and conscientiousness, one can intuitively infer their propensity to replicate the same behaviour in their daily practice and, thus, contribute to their anxiety level. This is an example of the influence of "medical culture" on young physicians. This characteristic is a perpetuated conduct in medical practice that is not constructive amongst clinicians. Furthermore, this "cultural" pressure in which doctors work daily gives further awareness to the physician-as-a-patient, who then elaborates a censored communication with their curer, extracting what they might think is useful or not useful information. Subsequently, this may trigger a series of wrong actions in making the correct diagnosis and prescribing an efficient treatment.

Compared with lay patients, doctors-as-patients do not exclusively rely on their physician's knowledge. Often, as proven previously, they are self-diagnosing and offer only what they consider essential from their symptomatology. In this case, the analogy with the Inga-otto thought experiment is difficult to realise. The reason is that the patient is not oblivious to the significance of their symptoms, possible treatment and the overall outcome. The degree of uncertainty depends mainly on the nature of the known medical condition and not necessarily on the informational load they possess.

In the case of a lay patient, they are physician resourced, and their doctor is brain resourced, like Otto was paper resourced, and Inga was brain resourced. On the other hand, the physician-as-patient does not rely exclusively on their doctor's knowledge but also theirs; they are, thus, both brain and physician resourced. Which of these resources is more dominant, brain or physician, depends on the physician-as-patient's choice. They may follow their brain-based resource, as Inga did to reach point B, and, at the same time, use the external resource, their physician's brain, to have their hypothesis regarding possible diagnosis validated—because they do not rely on other external resources but mainly on their memory.

> The doctor-patient usually thinks he knows the diagnosis, even if it is the wrong one. Ordinary patients have confidence in their physician's skill, but the medical training of physician-patients gets in their way. [12, p. 434].

If we follow this line of judgement, the physician is partially the cognitive extension of the physician-as-patient mind due to the control they automatically manifest regarding their condition. It is about how much power they allow their physician to exhibit.

Diagram 6.1. The physician–lay patient knowledge framework reflected the informational flow between the lay patient and the doctor. Compared with the situations where the patient is a physician or a medical-trained person, the diagram could change, as shown in Diagram 6.2, Lay patient—Physician knowledge framework and Diagram 6.3, Physician-as-patient—Physician knowledge framework

In Diagram 6.2, step 1 denotes the moment when the signs (indirect) and symptoms (from direct communication) coming from the lay patient are integrated and processed further by the physician's mind. In contrast, in Diagram 6.3, step 1 reflects the physician-as-patients presenting the symptoms to the physician after filtering them to make a specific case; the signs are the least filtered information, since they cannot be hidden. Therefore, the attending physician has limited access to the subjective part of the physician-as-patient illness, their symptomatology. At the same time, the latter is still the one who can control the informational load they choose to present or not. From this perspective, the power ratio between the two is different

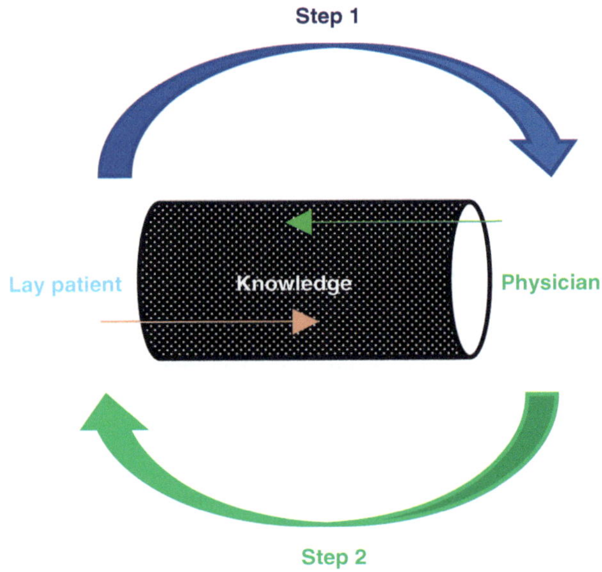

Diagram 6.2 Lay patient—Physician knowledge framework

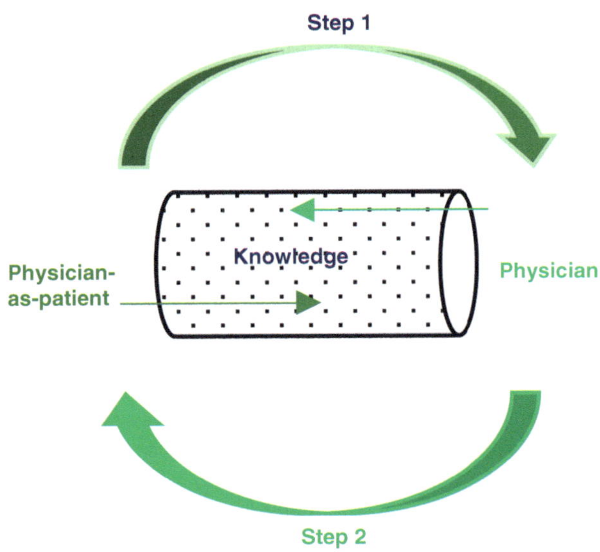

Diagram 6.3 Physician-as-patient—Physician knowledge framework

than expected (see Chap. 2 Gaps in Understanding the Doctor-Patient Relationship.), since the physician-as-patient is in greater control than the lay patient.

In Diagram 6.2, step 2 reflects the informational exchange between the physician and the lay patient, which appears to be more accessible than the physician-as-patients due to their control in this process. This process includes all other underlying mechanisms that manifest with the downfall from the position of power to that of disempowerment, as presented previously—the downfall from being a doctor to being a patient.

Therefore, contrary to the lay patient-physician rapport, the physician of the physician-as-patient (PAP) does not represent the latter's extension of their mind. The PAP does not entirely depend on the attendant physician's (AP) knowledge and not even on their authority. The AP, nevertheless, relies on their scientific (knowledge-based) and implicit (experience-based) information, which they retrieve from their memory. Although the data coming from the AP equals the information that Otto needs to reach point B by accessing them from the notebook, the PAP may be oblivious to this information if they consider they know better what they suffer from or what the best treatment may be for them. Thus, PAP is not Otto's homologous, because they have direct access to that information and do not need external resources—PAP is brain resourced, while the lay patient is physician resourced—unless the PAP recognises the AP's role by accepting their new position, that of a patient and not remaining in the role they were used to in their profession.

The conclusions that can follow from these two cases is that the patient's mind is extended to the physician (1) entirely if the patient is a layperson or a medical professional who accepts the role of a patient or (2) partially if the patient considered knows better than their attending physician.

References

1. Clark A, Chalmers D (1998) The extended mind. Analysis 58:7–19. https://doi.org/10.1093/analys/58.1.7
2. Aizawa K (2015) Extended cognition. In: The Routledge handbook of embodied cognition. https://doi.org/10.4324/9781315775845.ch3
3. Menary R (2010) The extended mind. MIT, Cambridge, MA
4. Shapiro L (2014) Extended cognition. In: The Routledge handbook of embodied cognition. Routledge, pp 31–38
5. Clark A (2010) Memento's revenge: the extended mind, extended. In: The extended mind. The MIT Press, pp 43–66
6. Aizawa K (2014) Extended cognition. In: The Routledge handbook of embodied cognition. Routledge, pp 31–38
7. Benedetti F (2011) Seeking relief: the activation of motivational and reward circuits. In: Benedetti F (ed) The patient's brain: the neuroscience behind the doctor-patient relationship. Oxford University Press, Oxford, pp 101–122
8. Zadra JR, Clore GL (2011) Emotion and perception: the role of affective information. Wiley Interdiscip Rev Cogn Sci 2:676–685
9. Derryberry D, Tucker DM (1994) Motivating the focus of attention. In: Niedenthal PM, Shinobu K (eds) The heart's eye: emotional influences in perception and attention. Academic, pp 167–196
10. Fredrickson BL (2004) The broaden–and–build theory of positive emotions. Philos Trans R Soc Lond Ser B Biol Sci 359:1367–1377
11. Myers MF, Gabbard GO (2008) The physician as patient. A clinical handbook for mental health professionals. American Psychiatric Publishing, Arlington
12. Mandell H, Spiro H (1988) When doctors get sick. https://doi.org/10.1007/978-1-4899-2001-0
13. Jenkins JF (1896) The physician as a patient. J Am Med Assoc XXVII:1166
14. Hahn RA (1985) Between two worlds physicians as patients. Med Anthropol Q 16:87–98
15. Sacks O (2020) A leg to stand on. Vintage. Reprint edition

16. Marcum JA (2008) An introductory philosophy of medicine. Humanizing modern medicine. https://doi.org/10.1007/978-1-4020-6797-6
17. Beevers CG, Miller IW (2004) Perfectionism, cognitive bias, and hopelessness as prospective predictors of suicidal ideation. Suicide Life Threat Behav 34:126–137
18. Hamilton TK, Schweitzer RD (2000) The cost of being perfect: perfectionism and suicide ideation in university students. Aust N Z J Psychiatry 34:829–835

Chapter 7
Placebo: Evidence of the Patient's Extended Mind

7.1 Introduction

From a scientific perspective, the complexity of the patient-doctor relationship can be understood mainly through objective and observational placebo findings. Therefore, throughout this chapter, subjective and objective considerations of the placebo effect and response are treated as distinctive terms. To make specific correlations between the placebo mechanisms and their implications as key factors in advancing the extended mind theory within the medical environment, I must first clarify the meaning of the words used in this context.

Since the beginning of its usage, the meaning of "placebo" changed repeatedly. It was first used in Latin.[1] Around the fourteenth century, it had a profane sense[2] [1, pp. 717–728], whilst, in the eighteenth century, the imposters used "placebo substances" to mislead patients. In the twentieth century, it was considered a cornerstone for medical research in randomised control trials[3] [2, p. 125]. In the past decades, "placebo" has been used in a broader sense, extending the underlying generating factors from substances-involved placebo, "pure"[4] or "impure"[5] placebo [3], to non-substances-involved placebo, namely, the physician-patient interaction through the therapeutical ritual [4].

---

[1] "To please" [1, p. 2].

[2] "Singing the Psalm 116" by "professional mourners (…) as cunning flatterers" in the Catholic church around the fourteenth century" [1, p. 3].

[3] "A necessary background 'noise' that must be subtracted from the results on a trial" [1, p. 4].

[4] "Pure placebos are interventions such as sugar pills or saline injections without direct pharmacologically active ingredients for the condition being treated" [3, p. 2] .

[5] "substances, interventions or 'therapeutic' methods which have known pharmacological, clinical or physical value for some ailments but lack specific therapeutic effects or value for the condition for which they have been prescribed" [ibid.].

G.-P. Florea, *Metacognition and Medical Humanities in Medical Education*, New Paradigms in Healthcare, https://doi.org/10.1007/978-3-032-01070-4_7

The placebo's translation from Latin is "I shall please" and is often used interchangeably with the term "sham," which means "a trick that deludes" [5], referring to fake procedures like sham surgery or sham acupuncture treatments.

According to Taber's Cyclopedic Medical Dictionary [6], placebo has two meanings: (1) "an inactive substance or treatment given instead of one that has proven effects" and (2) "drug or treatment used in non-specific or inactive control in a test of a therapy that is suspected of being useful for a particular disease or condition" [6, p. 1831]. Moreover, *placebo* is the generical word for the phenomenon, whilst the "placebo effect" offers the biopsychological perspective of its complex effect [7, pp. 407–8].

Since the early stages of discovering the existence of induced alleviation of symptoms [8, 9], the so-called placebo, consistent progress has been made. In those days and initial stages, the word placebo was attributed only to sham therapies or treatments. Currently, a placebo plays a crucial role when evaluating the efficacy of an active substance or intervention in the randomised, double-blind placebo-controlled clinical trial (RDBPC), a gold standard in modern clinical research: it has a (1) randomisation component, because the intervention is assigned arbitrarily, (2) double-blind factor, because neither the investigator nor the person that takes part in that study knows whether or not the applied treatment is actual (active) or fake (placebo)—and (3) placebo control group, because the trial has two, or more groups, of which one is receiving the active substance and another an inactive one (the placebo group) for the results to be compared after that. This experimental study is considered valuable, because it eliminates the biases based on expectations, also known as "therapeutical bias," since both involved are blinded. Thus, it reduces the incorrect estimation of the effect of the treatment under investigation. From Miro Jakovljevic's perspective, these considerations are devalued, arguing that clinical trials are based on various myths [10, p. 334].

The primary purpose is to use placebos to investigate an active substance's efficacy within in vitro conditions.[6] On the other hand, in vivo, in the same context, would introduce new parameters within clinical research that include social and psychological traits alongside biological and genetic ones. Following Jakovljevic, these myths are at the core of modern research protocols. They are neither more nor less than biases within the fundament of medical research reasoning, because research based on placebo biases determines "impure" results and observations. With the specificity of using a placebo, the RDBPCs reveal an understanding of the patient's mind and its implication in their overall health outcome.

In the past decades, the neurobiological effect (and response) that a placebo has in clinical practice has been described through empirical studies. Many scholars have proved that a "placebo approach" used in clinical trials is more than a method for demonstrating a drug's chemical effect in humans [11–16]. Fabrizio Benedetti [4, 12, 13, 17–20] and Ted J Kaptchuk [20–22] were two of the fewest scientists

[6] In this context, in vitro means taking the person away from their personal context and the outer milieu with which they exchange mental and emotional information translated within the body by biochemical and physiological reactions that determine physical and behavioural changes.

conducting essential studies on the neuroscience behind the doctor-patient relationship. Moreover, Benedetti et al. [23] emphasise the importance of the doctor-patient interaction, since the inert substances that constitute the placebo are not therapeutical [23 p. 339]. Price et al. attribute the placebo phenomenon to "environmental and psychosocial determinants" like "verbal suggestions and behaviours manifested by healthcare providers" [19 p. 568].

Insofar as the specialised literature goes, a significant ambiguity is built around the placebo's semantic field. Whether some researchers [10, 24–27] clearly distinguish between placebo effect and placebo response, others [18, 28–31] use them interchangeably. Additionally, amongst the advocates of the former category, some bring into discussion conceptual understanding [10 p. 334, 26 p. 38] whilst others make an appeal to logic for distinguishing between them by referring to *post* and *propter hoc* placebo administration—"the placebo effect is the difference between the placebo response and the changes that would be observed even without the administration of a placebo [...] subtract changes due to the natural history of the disorder and regression toward the mean." [25, p. 102]. Wager and Fields emphasize the difference between response and effect for that the effect is "an active neurobiological process that occurs as a result of placebo treatment," whilst the response expresses the "observable differences" between two groups from a clinical trial, one that received a placebo and the other that did not receive any treatment, "attributable to the efficacy of the placebo" [24, p. 363]. In addition, Evers et al. add to this core definition the disease's natural regression to the mean,[7] and describing the placebo effect as the "neurobiological and psychological mechanisms of expectancies" [20, p. 206]. Richard Kradin, on the other hand, defines placebo response as "(1) a complex mind–body interaction (2) evoked within a therapeutic dynamic, in which (3) the offer to treat (4) a pre-existing dysphoric condition with (5) an inert or ineffective intervention (i.e., a placebo) (6) results in the restoration of well-being," whereas the placebo effect as "the subjective feeling of well-being" [26 p. 38]. For a concise overview of the differences between effects and responses in placebo research, see Table 7.1.

Whether I choose to use the placebo effect as distinct from the placebo response may be irrelevant, since conscious or unconscious mental processes are at the core of this phenomenon. However, I chose not to use them interchangeably but to start from the fact that the "placebo response" implies all changes within the health status of a patient after receiving a placebo, changes that are embedded within the "placebo effect": the neurophysiological and psychological changes due to various sets of belief and expectation. By accepting this premise, when talking about placebo response, the existence of a placebo effect cannot be disputed, let alone its "psychosocial context effect (...) that different social stimuli, such as words and rituals of the therapeutic act, may change the chemistry and circuitry of the patient's brain" [32].

[7] "Regression to the mean or regression towards the mean is "the likelihood that over time probable events will occur and a normal distribution of events rather than that rare, unlikely, or unusual events will unfold" [6].

Table 7.1 Differences between effects and responses in placebo research

Notion	Meaning
Placebo	"An inactive substance substituted for a drug or a meaningless treatment substituted for an experimental treatment given to a control group during an experiment to prevent subjects and, sometimes, the experimenter from knowing they did not receive the treatment so they can be used as a comparison group for the group that received the treatment." [7 p. 388]
Also knows as	*Sugar pill, dummy treatment, inert/inactive/non-specific substance/treatment with respect to particular clinical outcomes.*
Placebo effect	A neurobiological process triggered by a placebo-objective determination
Treatment effect	The actual effect of an active substance/treatment, including the contextual effects.
Also referred to as	*Efficacy*
Placebo response	"The change in functioning or behavior brought about by administering an inert substance or non-specific treatment seems to be caused by a belief that a subject has received treatment." [7, p. 389]; A series of effects (so-called noises) that have to be differentiated by specific treatment efficacy—subjective
Also referred to as	*Contextual effects*
Placebo reactor/ placebo responder	A person who reacts or responds positively to a neutral or inactive treatment or intervention [9, p. 1602]

Although each research group identified (or not) relevant peculiarities within the mechanism involved in delivering placebos, a consensus regarding its importance and the underlying mechanisms has been emphasised.

7.2 The Placebo Effect and Its Neurological Response: Implications on Perception and Behaviour

In the past decade, many empirical studies have described a placebo's neurobiological effect or response in clinical practice. Many scholars have proved that a "placebo approach" used in clinical trials is more than a method for demonstrating a drug's chemical effect in humans [11–16].

7.2.1 *Placebo and Perception*

The list of keywords includes nociception and nociceptors, the sensory-discriminative system, the cognitive-affective system, top-down and bottom-up modulation, placebo, the placebo effect and placebo response.

Nociception[8] describes the body's ability to detect painful stimuli (extreme heat, cold, mechanical and chemical signals) by passing this information through the peripheral and central nervous system's structures [33]. The end effect is an action potential translated into a reflexive response. A typical example of such a response is one's reaction when reaching a heated surface: the person will retract immediately that part of the body that came in contact with the painful (heat) stimulus.

Nociceptors are cutaneous or subcutaneous sensory receptors signalling the presence of noxious stimuli. In other words, they are receptors for painful stimuli. Noxious, harmful stimuli activate nociceptors and elicit tissue damage.

Top-down or descending modulation is a subject-driven cortical mechanism associated with attention. In contrast, bottom-up modulation is a stimulus-driven cortical mechanism of attentional pain modulation associated with stimulus intensity [34].

The sensory-discriminative system is related to pain's intensity or sensorial aspect, including its spatial and temporal qualitative features [35].

The cognitive-affective system is a theory meant to explain human variations and disposition differences. It relates to the "If ... Then...." [36, pp. 248–50] statements on building thinking and behaviour patterns—see Fig. 7.1.

If, until recently, pain processing was attributed to the sensory-discriminative and cognitive-affective systems, nowadays, this theory is no longer valid. The sensory-discriminative system was thought to be involved in processing nociceptive input (e.g., pain's location, intensity, and quality). In contrast, the cognitive-affective system is the psychological aspect of the pain. Eventually, it was proven that brain regions of the sensory-discriminative[9] system could respond to mental processes like brain regions involved in the cognitive-affective system[10] do [35]. Moreover, advanced studies [24, 37] achieved higher predictability when both regions were considered. Therefore, when brain mapping the "neurological pain signature," regions[11] from both systems were highlighted when healthy volunteer subjects were experiencing induced heat pain [37].

7.2.2 *Placebo and Behaviour*

According to Benedetti et al., the evidence of a biological system that triggers a specific behaviour in patients seeking clinical amelioration comes mainly from placebo research [23]. The mesolimbic dopaminergic system was found to be activated

[8] *noci-* the Latin prefix denoting pain.

[9] The lateral thalamus and primary and secondary somatosensory cortex.

[10] The anterior insula and anterior cingulate cortex.

[11] Thalamus, primary and secondary somatosensory cortex, anterior insula and anterior cingulate cortex [37].

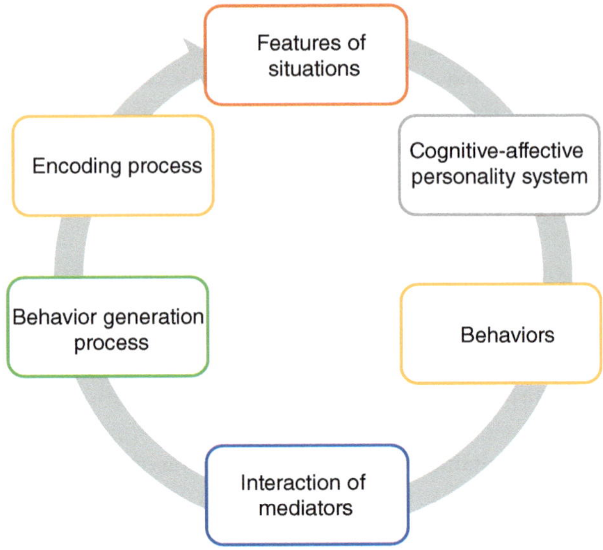

Fig. 7.1 Cognitive-affective system theory of personality. (Adapted from Mischel and Shoda [36])

in some medical conditions[12] when expecting clinical improvement [4]. Benedetti distinguishes between the behaviour of seeking relief and the behaviour of seeking pleasure. For instance, sex, self-administration of drugs or abuse, and gambling work on a reward and seeking pleasure mechanism, whilst seeking relief is a motivational behaviour to suppress discomfort. This behaviour is compared with the person's survival mechanism based on motivations like hunger, thirst or thermoregulation. If the behaviour based on reward does not cause any harm, seeking pain relief, in our case, when medical care is lacking, is as harmful as the lack of food or water in hunger or thirst. The distinction between suppressing discomfort and seeking pleasure by getting a reward can have a similar outcome. At a biological level, the underlying mechanism involves "the mesolimbic dopaminergic system: the ventral tegmental area, the nucleus accumbens, and the prefrontal cortex" (ibid.). Following this pathway, Benedetti assumes that the patient first relies "on the healer who, he believes, is capable of suppressing the pathological process" [32, p. 102]. Benedetti concludes that "[b]y considering the sickness-suppressing-motivated behaviour and the involvement of the motivation/reward neural network, the clinician must consider himself a powerful reward; thus, any effort should be directed to enhance the reward mechanisms. It will become clear (…) that therapy can, at least in some circumstances, be conceptualised as a reward" [ibid.].

Generically speaking, feeling sick is "an intricate combination of bottom-up and top-down events that eventually initiates the seeking behaviour aimed at suppressing both physical discomfort and negative emotions" [32, p. 53]. The perception of being sick is due to the interoceptive sensibility of each person, triggered by specific receptors found in cortical and subcortical regions involved in awareness

[12] "In at least three medical conditions, like Parkinson's disease, depression and pain" [4, p. 102].

processing, "the insular cortex and the anterior cingulate cortex" [ibid.]. Some emotional states contribute to these cortex areas' capacity to manifest awareness of being sick. Because of this, "perceptions can be reported in different ways from time to time, and interoceptive-evoked brain activity may vary in different circumstances" [38, p. 53]. It means that emotions like fear, anxiety, and cognitive tasks (involving attention and distraction) may modulate the feeling of being sick. Negative emotions are essential in "feeling sick because they modulate the magnitude of a symptom, e.g., pain" [38, p. 54].

7.3 Where Does the Extension of a Patient's Mind Begin, and Where Does It End? The Auxiliary Cortex Theory

The answer to the question "Where does the extension of a patient's mind begin, and where does it end?" relates to Clark and Chalmers' theory of the extended mind transposed to the medical environment to endorse the cognitive coupling system argument in the doctor-patient relationship, presented previously. Also, the neuroscience within the patient-doctor relationship demonstrates the dependent relationship between the patient and the doctor, as proven in Sect. 7.2. The Placebo Effect and its Neurological Response: Implications on Perception and Behaviour. For further emphasis, in the last part of this chapter, an add-on to the view that shows the neurobiological changes that occur in the doctor-patient relationship is presented through Salvador's theory regarding the auxiliary cortex [39].

From a fundamental perspective, there may not be a more straightforward way to look at the doctor-patient relationship than comparing it with the relationship between a mother and their newborn. It is needless to assert that an infant is *tabula rasa* when it comes to anything that life offers from either the physical or mental dimension. In the early stages of their development, a child relies mainly on their mother regarding primary needs like food, physiological advances such as locomotion or speaking, and secondary growth aspects, including communicating and expressing themselves emotionally through mimicry. The mother is there to provide food for her child for physical development, to support and encourage the act of walking in the stage of neurons' myelinisation involved in the locomotion progress, to help in developing communication abilities in an articulated and coherent manner, and last but not least to nurture emotional answer and exchange emotional responses. In these lines of thought, Salvador posits that a mother acts like a child's "auxiliary cortex" in the first months of age [39, p. 43]. He sets some rules psychotherapists should follow, one of which is to "act as an "external auxiliary cortex"" for a patient. Even though a physician is not a psychotherapist for a patient, the medical condition can determine mental and emotional distress due to the emotional charge added to the physical ailment.

Additionally, following Clark and Chalmers' claim: "We advocate a very different sort of externalism: an active externalism, based on the active role of the environment in driving cognitive processes" [40, p. 7], I consider that the doctor-patient relationship is a form of *active externalism*. Furthermore, Benedetti et al. claimed that the mechanism behind placebo is not visible, because research studies aim to see if "drugs are better than placebos" [23, p. 339] whilst the interaction through the therapeutical ritual within the doctor-patient interaction is what determines the placebo effect, and not the inactive substance itself. From a neuroscience point of view, they imply that the physician is seen through the patient's eye lenses as a saviour to whom they can manifest their fragility and cry for help [23, p. 102].

Therefore, Salvador's and Benedetti's views, taken in conjunction, can constitute the solid argument that mentally, the patient does look at the physician as "God almighty," and the doctor may even be empowered by them as such, even if not consciously. Consequently, the patient knowingly or unconsciously expects some profound moral and trustworthy practice principles to rely on their physician. In this sense, I claim that Salvador's view should be considered equally important in the physician-patient relationship, since the physician can be seen as the patient's external auxiliary cortex.

Applying Clark and Chalmers' EMT to the medical context, the physician can represent the patient's extended mind. Also, from Salvador's perspective, the conclusion that physicians play the role of a patient's "external auxiliary cortex" as a mother does for her child by identifying and meeting the patient's needs, "calming him and intervening in his welfare, and creating homeostasis" [39, p. 43] can be drawn.

After discussing in detail, the typologies that patients and medical professionals can ascribe, one could identify a different category of patients, as laypeople or physicians-as-patients; moreover, a further division could be recognised even between them. We have seen that each of these categories commonly assumes the fear of the unknown for lay patients, or the known for physicians-as-patients, and the fear of death for all sorts of patients. Because physicians-as-patients have a more complex and holistic understanding of the concept of disease, in its wholeness—possible implications and complications—and what their physicians may temporarily omit to say to protect them—the internal stress level may be significant in all cases. Even though, at first glance, it may seem that a physician is a better-informed patient due to the experience-based knowledge in medical practice, this very fact represents a disadvantage in the therapeutical process and not a benefit.

The question I raised: "Where does the extension of the patient's mind begin and where does it end?" can be easy and challenging to answer simultaneously. It is easy if we choose the simple answer: there is not a beginning nor an end to it, because the participants in the medical act are in a continuous *modus operandi*; the situation in which the patient finds themselves is as equally simple as complex according to their depth in knowledge or emotion in the realm of the known versus unknown elements accompanying the medical condition, and their implication in the inherent fear of death. At the same time, the answer can be complex if we consider both inputs, the patient's and the physician's, coming from beings with an intricate understanding of health, disease, illness, life and/or death.

The fact that the patient relies on the physician's mind is easy to accept, since they cannot retrieve the medical information from a notebook, as Otto does. Nevertheless, mentally reliable patients' memories, either lay patient or physician-as-a-patient, as altered as they get based on the positive or negative emotion charge of the moment of receiving the diagnosis, play the same role as the data stored in Otto's notebook. The objection one may raise here is the information alteration Otto holds within the notebook, since it may amplify or narrow down his perception of the medical condition.

7.4 Discussion

The EMT applied in a medical context could endorse the patient's mind extended into the clinical setting, hence the justification of the neurobiological changes behind a placebo determined by the therapeutical ritual. Therefore, in extenso, this correlation endorses the philosophical perspective about the EMT and, at the same time, emphasises the physician's mental *capacity* to diagnose, treat and care for the patient. Both perspectives also imply the necessity for the *ability* to care for the patient using a compassionate care approach as an add-on to the formal clinical guidelines. I use the term *ability* to express a physician's strength, be it mental, emotional, inborn, or gained, and the *capacity* to convey the potential of enhancing that ability. I distinguish between the ability and the capacity to show passionate care depending on the physician's resources and the patient's needs.

The placebo effect is based on the "patient's needs, personality, psychological state, genetics, the severity and discomfort of the symptoms, the type of verbal instructions, the preparation characteristics, and the environment milieu" [18, p. 1208] but not least, the patient's as well as doctor's expectations. These alone suggest the patient's unicity and the physician's capacity to treat the patient as a holistic individual and not in a frame of mind based on the principle of a statistical cohort of people with the same characteristics. This aspect emphasises the need to develop or enhance social skills in future doctors, including verbal and nonverbal communication. Consequently, it implies a proper therapeutic ritual tailored to each individual needing medical support.

In short, the patient-physician relationship is a connection created amongst the medical agent, the doctor and the ill person, the patient. Their relationship revolves around the physiological dysfunction(s) the patient suffers from. The doctor aims to seek medical solutions to improve a patient's health status and/or prevent a new disease that can pile up from the initial one. Hence, the physician treats the active disease and prevents the appearance of a new one. There is, of course, another possibility in the case of a dying patient where curing is not possible and where the aim is to make the process as painless as possible.

7.5 Conclusion

Through the lens of the philosophy of mind applied to the doctor-patient relationship, it is clear that the interplay between cognition and medical practice underscores the significance of cognitive processes in understanding the nuances of the doctor-patient dynamic, particularly through the lens of the Extended Mind Theory (EMT) and the placebo effect. By examining the cognitive coupling between patient and physician, this chapter explains how this relationship extends beyond mere interaction to form a coupling cognitive system, significantly influencing patient outcomes.

The arguments are based on the placebo mechanism, showing its relevance in clinical trials and the dynamics of the doctor-patient interaction. In this context, the placebo effect is not a mere byproduct of randomised control trials but a crucial element that reflects the intertwined nature of mind, body and the therapeutic environment. The chapter articulates how a physician's actions and the therapeutic setting activate neurobiological responses in patients, thus extending the patient's mind into the medical environment and vice versa. Henceforth, the placebo response is the patient's physical manifestation and mental expression, which triggers neurobiological objectifiable changes for the individual subject to medical intervention, the placebo effect. In other words, the placebo effect is the embodiment, as well as the extension into the world, of the placebo response.

Furthermore, the analysis of the patient-physician rapport as a cognitive coupling system offers insights into how the individual mental states of both doctor and patient influence and are influenced by their interaction; it is not a one-way street but a complex, dynamic process that contributes significantly to the therapeutic outcome. The theory of the physician as an "auxiliary cortex" to the patient further enriches this discussion, presenting the physician's role as not only a doctor but also a critical extension of the patient's cognitive and emotional processing.

The philosophical perspective, particularly through the Extended Mind Theory and the concept of the physician as an auxiliary cortex, provides a novel lens through which to view and improve the therapeutic alliance. Acknowledging these conceptual tools in the medical setting could offer a valuable perspective, highlighting the significant role that physicians play in shaping patient outcomes. Therefore, as we move forward, medical practitioners and philosophers of mind must continue exploring these connections for a more holistic approach to healthcare that recognises the intricate interplay amongst mind, body and environment.

References

1. Louhiala P, Puustinen R (2017) Meaning and use of placebo: philosophical considerations. In: Schramme T, Edwards S (eds) Handbook of the philosophy of medicine. Springer, Dordrecht, pp 1–12
2. Hunter P (2007) A question of faith. EMBO Rep 8:125–128

3. Howick J, Bishop FL, Heneghan C, Wolstenholme J, Stevens S, Hobbs FDR, Lewith G (2013) Placebo use in the United Kingdom: results from a national survey of primary care practitioners. PLoS One. https://doi.org/10.1371/journal.pone.0058247
4. Benedetti F (2011) The patient's brain: the neuroscience behind the doctor-patient relationship. Oxford University Press
5. Sham definition & meaning—Merriam-Webster. 2022; https://www.merriam-webster.com/dictionary/sham. Accessed 5 July 2022
6. Venes D (2017) Taber's Cyclopedic medical dictionary, 23rd edn. F.A. Davis Company
7. Matsumoto D (2009) The Cambridge dictionary of psychology. Cambridge University Press
8. Haygarth J (1800) Literary and philosophical Society of Bath. In: Of the imagination as a cause and cure of disorders of the body; exemplified by fictitious tractors. Cruttwell, Bath, pp 133–145
9. Beecher HK (1955) The powerful placebo. JAMA J Am Med Assoc 159:1602–1606
10. Jakovljevic M (2013) The placebo-nocebo response: controversies and challenges from clinical and research perspective. Eur Neuropsychopharmacol 24:333–341
11. Brody H, Waters DB (1980) Diagnosis is treatment. J Fam Pract 10:445–449
12. Benedetti F (2002) How the doctor's words affect the patient's brain. Eval Health Prof 25:369–386
13. Benedetti F, Maggi G, Lopiano L, Lanotte M, Rainero I, Vighetti S, Pollo A (2003) Open versus hidden medical treatments: the patient's knowledge about a therapy affects the therapy outcome. Prev Treat. https://doi.org/10.1037/1522-3736.6.1.61a
14. Thompson JJ, Ritenbaugh C, Nichter M (2009) Reconsidering the placebo response from a broad anthropological perspective. Cult Med Psychiatry 33:112–152
15. Wiech K (1979) (2016) deconstructing the sensation of pain: the influence of cognitive processes on pain perception. Science 354:584–587
16. Ongaro G, Kaptchuk TJ (2019) Symptom perception, placebo effects, and the Bayesian brain. Pain 160:1–4
17. Benedetti F (2016) Placebo effects—understanding the mechanisms in health and disease. Physiosciene 12
18. Benedetti F (2013) Placebo and the new physiology of the doctor-patient relationship. Physiol Rev 93:1207–1246
19. Price DD, Finniss DG, Benedetti F (2008) A comprehensive review of the placebo effect: recent advances and current thought. Annu Rev Psychol 59:565–590
20. Evers AWM, Colloca L, Blease C et al (2018) Implications of placebo and nocebo effects for clinical practice: expert consensus. Psychother Psychosom 87:204–210
21. Kaptchuk TJ (2018) Open-label placebo: reflections on a research agenda. Perspect Biol Med 61:311–334
22. Kaptchuk TJ, Miller FG (2018) Open label placebo: can honestly prescribed placebos evoke meaningful therapeutic benefits? Br Med J. https://doi.org/10.1136/bmj.k3889
23. Benedetti F, Carlino E, Pollo A (2011) How placebos change the patient's brain. Neuropsychopharmacology 36:339–354
24. Wager TD, Fields HL (2013) Placebo Analgesia. In: McMahon SB, Koltzenburg M, Tracey I, Turk D (eds) Wall and Melzack's textbook of pain. Elsevier Ltd, 6, pp 362–373
25. Kirsch I (2013) The placebo effect revisited: lessons learned to date. Complement Ther Med 21:102–104
26. Kradin RL (2010) Placebo response: a consideration of its role in therapeutics. Curr Psychiatry Rep 13:37–42
27. Hafliðadóttir SH, Juhl CB, Nielsen SM, Henriksen M, Harris IA, Bliddal H, Christensen R (2021) Placebo response and effect in randomized clinical trials: meta-research with focus on contextual effects. Trials 22:1–15
28. Buchanan WW, Bellamy N (1997) The placebo response: clinical efficacy and toxicity. In: Side effects of anti-inflammatory drugs IV. Kluwer Academic Publishers, London, pp 11–23
29. Kaptchuk TJ, Miller FG (2015) Placebo effects in medicine. N Engl J Med 373:8–9

30. Barrett B, Muller D, Rakel D, Rabago D, Marchand L, Scheder JC (2006) Placebo, meaning, and health. Perspect Biol Med 49:178–198
31. Geuter S, Koban L, Wager TD (2017) The cognitive neuroscience of placebo effects: concepts, predictions, and physiology. Annu Rev Neurosci 40:167–188
32. Benedetti F (2011) Seeking relief: the activation of motivational and reward circuits. In: Benedetti F (ed) The patient's brain: the neuroscience behind the doctor-patient relationship. Oxford University Press, pp 101–122
33. Rosenberg RN, Pascual JM (2014) Rosenberg's molecular and genetic basis of neurological and psychiatric disease, 5th edn. Elsevier
34. Hauck M, Domnick C, Lorenz J, Gerloff C, Engel AK (2015) Top-down and bottom-up modulation of pain-induced oscillations. Front Hum Neurosci 9:1–8
35. Auvray M, Myin E, Spence C (2010) The sensory-discriminative and affective-motivational aspects of pain. Neurosci Biobehav Rev. https://doi.org/10.1016/j.neubiorev.2008.07.008
36. Mischel W, Shoda Y (1995) A cognitive-affective system theory of personality: Reconceptualizing situations, dispositions, dynamics, and invariance in personality structure. Psychol Rev 102:246–268
37. Wager TD, Atlas LY, Lindquist MA, Roy M, Woo CW, Kross E (2013) An fMRI-based neurologic signature of physical pain. N Engl J Med 368:1388–1397
38. Benedetti F (2010) Feeling sick: a combination of bottom-up and top-down events. In: The patient's brain. Oxford University Press, pp 53–100
39. Salvador MC (2013) The wisdom of the subcortical brain. Int J Integr Psychother 4:40–53
40. Clark A, Chalmers D (1998) The extended mind. Analysis. https://doi.org/10.1093/analys/58.1.7

Part III
On Metacognition and Medicine

Chapter 8
Metacognition from A to Z and Its Relevance in Medicine

8.1 Introduction

Philosophers of medicine and medical researchers have made significant progress in tackling various sensitive aspects regarding the distinction between object and subject or disease and sufferance [1–3], the analysis of medical language [4], clinical reasoning and judgement, or medical decision making [4–11], the metacognitive component in medical rationale [12], autonomy in the doctor-patient relationship [13, 14], mind-body dualism, the biomedical model, and the biopsychosocial model or reductionism versus holism in medicine [15–22], virtues in medical practice [23], uncertainty in medicine [24] and many others. The cognitive involvement of patients in their treatment has been examined through studies on the placebo and nocebo effects [25–30]—see Sect. 7.2 The Placebo Effect and its Neurological Response: Implications on Perception and Behaviour. However, doctors' cognitive processes, particularly as they relate to their patients, have been explored in clinical decision making and not directly in terms of their relationship with the patient.

Physicians across all specialities encounter challenging scenarios in their practice. Patients' illness experiences are often intensely personal and may affect healthcare providers. Doctors deal with individuals who suffer from specific conditions and issues arising within the hospital's "medical society." Since physicians' *credo* and responsibility are to care for their patients, I claim they must become aware of their internal cognitive processes related to how their relationship with their patients affects them. This awareness is crucial for effectively navigating various situations in their relationships with the patient to benefit both parties. Thus, it is essential to

---

Fragments of this chapter have been published in Dumitru, Daniela, and Gabriela-Paula Florea. 2023. "The 'Irrational' Within Rational Thinking: Proofs from Medical Sciences and the Arts." In *Brain, Decision Making and Mental Health*, edited by Nima Rezaei, Integrated, 135–56. Springer Nature Switzerland. https://doi.org/10.1007/978-3-031-15959-6_8.

G.-P. Florea, *Metacognition and Medical Humanities in Medical Education*, New Paradigms in Healthcare, https://doi.org/10.1007/978-3-032-01070-4_8

examine the significance of their mental states: their direct thoughts and their awareness of these thoughts (object-level and meta-level cognition). Understanding these aspects is vital for (1) improving patient outcomes, (2) improving doctors' mental health and ultimately (3) enhancing their interaction.

8.2 The Interdisciplinary Debate on Metacognitive Thinking

In 1979, Flavell proposed a model for monitoring "cognitive enterprises." This model implies four types of phenomena, including "metacognitive knowledge," "metacognitive experiences," "goals or tasks" and "actions (or strategies)" [31, p. 906]. He defines metacognitive knowledge as the knowledge one stores intimately related to one's objectives (tasks, goals, actions or strategies) and experience, and metacognitive experience as the experience associated with the conscious or affective aspect of any mental process. The distinction he makes between these two and other cognitive processes relies only on the content or function and not on "form or quality" [ibid.].

According to Flavell, a segment of metacognitive knowledge can be activated intentionally or unintentionally. This activation "may and probably often does influence the course of the cognitive enterprise without itself entering consciousness" [ibid.]. Furthermore, this activation can lead to a "conscious experience" called a "metacognitive experience." Even though his primary research was on children in their developmental stages, Flavell suggests that these mental processes based on metacognitive knowledge "can have several concrete and important effects on the cognitive enterprises" of children and adults. He considers "overlapping sets" between metacognitive knowledge and metacognitive experiences and the effects of metacognitive experience on metacognitive knowledge by "adding to it, deleting from it, or revising it" [ibid.].

Over the past four decades, researchers in psychology developed various definitions for metacognition, from simple to more complex ones, depending on the attributes each research had been investigating.: "thinking about thinking," "cognition about cognitive phenomena" [ibid.], "cognition about cognition" [32, p. 2] or "set of capacities through which one operating cognitive subsystem is evaluated or represented by another in a context-sensitive way" [33, p. 29], amongst many. The difference relies on the epistemological perspective that one described. For instance Schneider and Lockl [34, p. 238] gave a more general definition, adding to the process of *cognition about cognition*, the "self-regulating processes that take cognitive processes as their object" when focussing on metacognitive knowledge in children and adolescents. On the other side of the spectrum, Hertzog offers a narrower definition of metacognition in gerontologic stages, introducing the property of memory's accuracy on self-reports in the elderly population [35, p. 169]. Koriat also gives a narrower definition as "people's cognitions and feelings about their cognitive states and cognitive processes" [36, p. 261]. Hertzog, thus, examines the implications of ageing on metacognitive processes, making it directly relevant to understanding changes in metacognition, particularly in older stages of life. At the same time, Schneider and Lockl centred their work on developing metacognitive knowledge in children and adolescents, emphasising early life stages. They offer a perspective on how self-evaluation is changing from early to older stages in life, showing that the young population overestimates its capacity to remember new information and, in contrast, the older population has a decreased confidence in this respect—it is about "memory self-efficacy," or one's appreciation concerning the capacity to remember new information, that these authors relate to. A graphical overview of metacognition's fields of research is represented through Diagram 8.1. The Epistemology of Metacognition. A visual representation of the various epistemological grounds on which metacognition stands, as a glimpse of its complexity across multiple research domains [37, p. 98].

Fleming and Frith assert that defining metacognition may lead one to confusion, because, nowadays, it carries different associations within an array of research fields like education, memory and perception [32]. They also stress the importance of the common fact, the "explicit conscious reflective awareness," because it

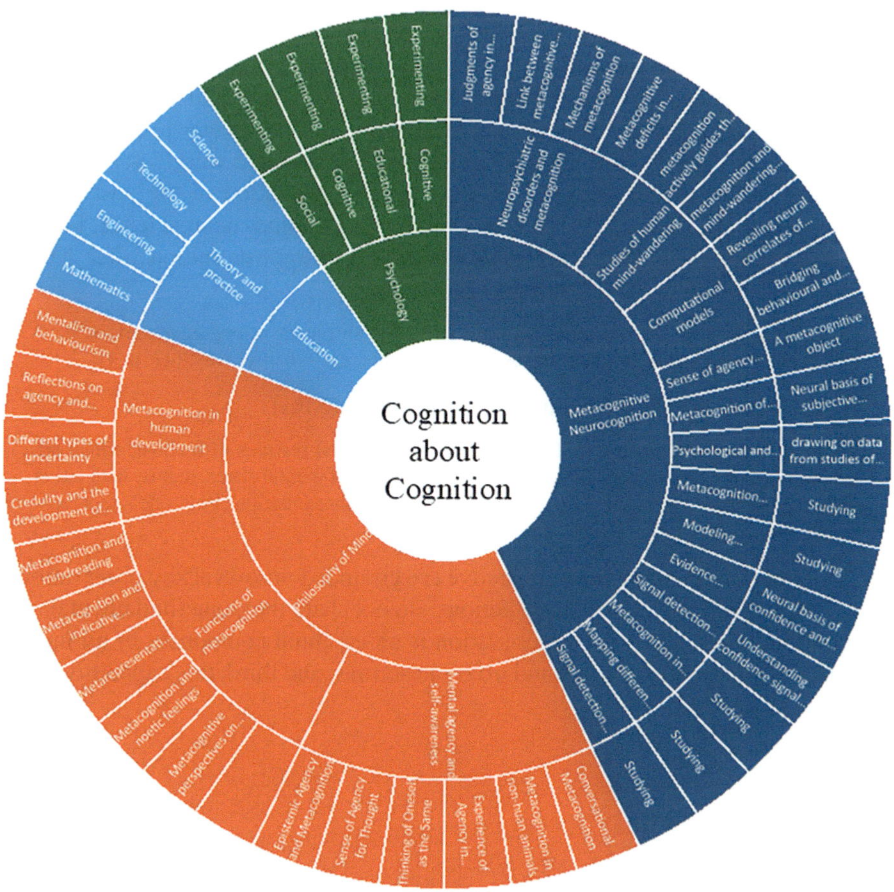

Diagram 8.1 The Epistemology of Metacognition. A visual representation of the various epistemological grounds on which metacognition stands, as a glimpse of its complexity in various research domains [1, p. 98]

"presents a barrier to a satisfactory computational and biological explanation of metacognition" [32, p. 2]. Therefore, they aim to fill in the biological gap by explaining the findings based on neuroscience.

In his meta-analysis regarding the most cited scholars until 2014, Dinsmore [38] identifies the top five researchers in psychology, developmental, educational and experimental psychology that came up with different theories and models of metacognition [31, 39–41]. He analysed the impact of ontological and epistemological groundings on the theories, models and methods chosen in metacognition research associated with self-regulation and self-learning based on Cartesian-split mechanistic tradition and the relational tradition framework. Akin to Fleming and Firth, Dinsmore pinpoints that instead of clarifying metacognition and its relation to self-regulation and self-learning, "the constructs and the relation between constructs became 'fuzzier'" [38, p. 1].

Later, in 1996, Nelson gathered philosophical and psychological approaches to metacognition's monitoring and controlling role [41]. He invokes Comte's Paradox of "how the brain can be both the organ being observed and the organ doing the observing," pointing out the difficulty of explaining the possibility of such phenomena' existence without the collaboration between psychologists and philosophers. He stresses the necessity of searching and building new models and theories, evoking the conceptual analysis of the possible worlds that can be a way to solve puzzles raised by consciousness through discovering "such a possible world" [41, p. 104].

Joelle Proust offers a complete and thorough explanation of the vast field of metacognition at a crossroads with the philosophy of mind, neuroscience, biology and psychology [42]. She gives a provisional "neutral" definition after having doubted the models proposed by other researchers:

> Metacognition is the set of capacities through which an operative cognitive subsystem is evaluated or represented by another subsystem in a context-sensitive way. [42, p. 4]

Also, Proust defends an exclusivist view, asserting that

> [M]etacognition is a natural kind: it has a set of functional features of its own, which are independent of those associated with the self-attribution of mental states, that is, with either self-directed mindreading or with other forms of metarepresentation about one's representations. [42, p. 5]

The assertions backing her perspective are grounded in several key observations: firstly, mental actions and ordinary actions[1] do not share the same fundamental normative framework; second, metacognition is an essential component of all mental actions, yet it is not present in standard basic actions; and third, this capability is not exclusive to humans.

[1] Physical movements.

8.3 What Is Metacognition?

The mental capacity to reflect on, monitor, evaluate and regulate one's own thinking processes carries the name of metacognition [31]. It is a complex skill set that relies on knowledge and experience regarding one's performance. This self-mental feature's effectiveness depends on the ability to regulate cognition based on past outcomes [43]. In other words, metacognition is a cognitive, inherent self-improvement mechanism that the human species developed and refined based on evolutionary precepts. As such, it may also be linked to our capacity to adapt or resile, depending on the situation.

This mental process of thinking about thinking requires mental skills that often come with specific embodied or affective feelings determining a metacognitive experience. On the one hand, the cognitive abilities on which metacognition is based are mental monitoring and evaluating the progress of one's task performance, as well as planning and controlling future strategies to enhance task efficiency. On the other hand, metacognitive processing can be experienced through bodily incorporation of metalevel mental processing like the Feeling of Knowing (FoK), the Feeling of Rightness (FoR) [44], or "gut feelings," a raw intuition trademark that will be addressed above. Another feeling associated with metacognition is the tip-of-the-tongue feeling or the temporary inaccessibility of a word predicated as a metacognitive experience [45].

Moreover, feelings with an affective load, thus perceived as mental states and not embodied, that relate to metacognition imply certain beliefs connected with the cognitive experience non-consciously and non-analytically derived. These metacognitive-related feelings are pivotal, since they ascend upon the process of cognition regulation through evaluation when pursuing a specific goal. They are related to the level of difficulty, satisfaction, confidence and familiarity with the task and determine an implicit attribution of qualitative features to reaching that objective. Therefore, they work on the motivational aspect of achieving the goal by measuring one's strengths and weaknesses and predicting success or failure. The decision to engage or disengage in starting, continuing, or not following the tasks is thus a result of perceiving one of these metacognitive, affective feelings essential for efficient work [43].

Metacognition encompasses fundamental processes and experiences that contribute to its twofold, conscious and unconscious, matrix: *metacognitive knowledge* (MK), *metacognitive experiences* (ME), *metacognitive regulation* (MR), as well as *metacognitive feelings* (MF) [31, 46–52]. MK reflects knowledge about one's cognitive ability, strategy, task or goal, whilst ME reflects those experiences related to conscious cognition and affection [31]. The "experienced-based metacognitive judgments" encompass the "feeling-of-knowing" and "tip-of-the-tongue" phenomena acting like intermediate stations or binders between the subconscious and conscious processes. This leads us to the fact that unconscious processes govern conscious feeling-of-knowing [46]. *Metacognitive regulation* (MR) involves cognitive monitoring as a bottom-up process and cognitive controlling as a top-down process [47]. It controls errors by *monitoring* them; it examines the source in the remembering process or assigns resources [52]; thus, it consciously coordinates cognition. Metacognitive reasoning based on knowledge uses explicit, analytic, conscious and controllable mental processes. Although *metacognitive feelings* (MFs) are linked to explicit, conscious cognition, a crossover view is also attached, since they mediate conscious and unconscious manners of action [53]. In other words, MK is based on explicit cognition, whilst MF manifests itself at the level of retrieving the implicit, unconscious mental processes towards the explicit, conscious ones [46].

Whilst in the early stage of understanding metacognitive processing, there was no evidence regarding the neural mechanisms involved, currently, we can rely on an increasing body of evidence. Cortex regions from the frontal (left supplementary motor area), prefrontal lobe (the inferior frontal gyrus, left opercular part), the parietal lobe (bilateral precuneus) or the limbic lobe (left dorsal anterior cingulate cortex) reveal activity in functional magnetic resonance imaging in subjects that monitor their or others' mental activity and actions [54–59]. Critchley et al. [60] found increased brain activity in several regions during an interoceptive task involving the timing of heartbeats. Significant activity was registered in the "insula, somatomotor cortex, supplementary motor area, and anterior cingulate cortex" [61]. Studies on emotional responses show a consistent co-activation pattern between the insular and anterior cingulate cortex, likely due to the dual projection of the lamina-1 spinothalamocortical tract to both regions [62]. It has been suggested that the anterior insular cortex plays a role in the experience of awareness. In contrast, the anterior cingulate cortex may be more closely linked to initiating behaviours [25]. Therefore, observing one's body and monitoring cognition triggers responses in common brain regions.

Even though all these cortex areas manifest significant responses in metacognitive processes, the dorsal anterior cingulate cortex (dACC) is the more complex one, both anatomically and functionally [63], due to its capacity to monitor and control cognitive and emotional processes. In short, dACC (1) monitors erroneous decision-making processes during or after making a decision [64], (2) monitors conflict between actions or strategies, (3) monitors reward (even if an essential number of studies did not prove a significant role in either negative or positive rewarding as other neurocognitive structures) and (4) possibly, it monitors fear and anxiety, though without significant evidence in human research [63].

According to Chris Frith [65], metacognition and its valence related to self-regulating cognition can be manifested implicitly or explicitly, where implicit implies involuntary, automatic, and explicit voluntary, hence mentally aware processing. Moreover, he brings forward this distinction of the human capacity to mentalise in social interaction. He asserts that humans' metacognitive ability to self-regulate is bidirectional, directed to self and others, which can be implicit or explicit. The essential key here concerns the ability to self-regulate mental processing through collective contribution. This true feature distinguishes us from other species that also manifest metacognitive processing, for example non-human primates such as Rhesus macaques [42]. Why is this important? Implicit metacognition is enacted in social interaction, and it enhances self-reflection through the process of mentalising or the process of thinking about another person's thinking. On the other hand, explicit metacognition is awareness of one's thinking process, enabling one to analyse and explain their actions to those around them.

8.3.1 The Working Definition of Metacognition

Although, as presented previously, metacognition was first introduced in psychology by the developmentalist John H. Flavell in 1979 [31], other related syntagms were mentioned even before, amongst which "memory-monitoring process," "tip-of-the-tongue experiences" or "feeling of knowing experiences" by Hart in 1965 [66]. Since then, the evolution of this concept has travelled many epistemological borders. Each field in which metacognition was investigated came with new research tools and methods, revealing its complexity. Due to differences of opinion and perspective, determining a unified theory is not possible. After Flavell [67] coined the term, other domains like neuroscience, philosophy of mind and psychiatry continued to raise new questions and claims about this mental phenomenon. Because metacognition seems "a many-headed monster" [39, p. 105], bringing together all the definitions and claims would inevitably deviate from the focus of this chapter's main aim.

Therefore, the working definition for metacognition used throughout the thesis is the explicit or implicit meta-level cognitive process that includes self-monitoring, self-evaluation, self-regulating and self-control of one's cognition, taken at the object level to achieve a specific goal, according to their roles and their own set of beliefs. Within a doctor-patient relationship, this definition envisages two perspectives, one of the physician's and the other of the patient's, following shared and individual goals. The goals that both parties share are the patient's best health outcomes and their improved quality of life. The personal goals depend on their roles and, additionally, on their set of beliefs with implications for their mental health. Thus, the difference resides in the strategies each needs to use to achieve these goals.

Therefore, from the physician's standpoint, metacognition is the implicit or explicit cognitive process of self-monitoring, self-evaluating, self-regulating and self-controlling their cognition with an effect on the clinical decision-making process and their relationship with the patient, impacting the patient's positive health outcome. Regarding the patient, metacognition is the patient's implicit or explicit cognitive process to self-monitor, self-evaluate, self-regulate and self-control their cognition with an effect on their positive health outcome, also influenced by the input resulting from the physician's approach. Although they both affect the medical interaction, the medical professional is the one that, by their professional *credo,* ought to also take into consideration the patient's cognitive input to obtain compliance with the treatment strategies.

8.4 Metacognition: An Indispensable Skill in the Doctor-Patient Relationship

A preliminary discussion concerning the necessity of introducing metacognitive models and methods into medical practice should include (a) the doctor's ability to recall information to elaborate a correct diagnosis, (b) the doctor's capacity for dealing with the patient's drama, not only with the object, that is the disease, (c) the patient as an active element (empowered) in the therapeutic process, (d) doctor-patient interaction and its effect on bringing positive changes within the patient's body, changes proven by Benedetti in the frame of doctor-patient interaction as a therapeutical ritual [25].

Firstly, bringing metacognition as a practical concept within the medical act would mean introducing new elements of cognitive skills as instruments that would need to be implemented by the doctor and the patient. The doctor would benefit by understanding how they retrieve memorised information [68] and adopting the approach according to the patient's needs. Secondly, the patient could internalise metacognitive knowledge through what Sodian et al. [69] called *collaborative conversations* with the doctor via metacognitive linguistic input; the patient would be part of their treatment process. Having in mind Flavell's model, proposing to monitor "cognitive enterprises" that are implying different phenomena,[2] a segment of metacognitive knowledge can be activated intentionally or unintentionally. Without relying on unintentional activation, the doctor can trigger this response in "collaborative conversations" as mentioned above. This intentional or unintentional activation "may and probably often does influence the course of the cognitive enterprise without itself entering consciousness" [31, p. 908], leading to the idea that patients experience this cognitive enterprise without themselves or their doctor being aware. This activation can lead to a "conscious experience" known as a "metacognitive experience." Because these mental processes based on metacognitive knowledge "can have several concrete and important effects on the cognitive enterprises" on children as well as on adults, activating intentional metacognitive expertise and bringing it to the level of metacognitive experience may lead the patient to positive effects on their healing process—as Benedetti indirectly asserts using a different epistemological framework [25]. Moreover, the doctor's role can be linked with Flavell's fifth assertion within the metacognitive model, which states the possibility of "overlapping sets" between metacognitive knowledge and metacognitive experiences and the effects that metacognition experience can have upon metacognitive knowledge by "adding to it, deleting from it, or revising it" [67, p. 908].

Nevertheless, one of the challenges may stem from the inability to fully integrate the diverse approaches to metacognition, preventing the formulation of a unifying theory. Metacognition's varied manifestations and applications make it complex, leading to overlapping yet distinct epistemological perspectives that extend beyond

[2] Metacognitive knowledge, goals/tasks and actions/strategies.

common ground. They intertwine because of the complexity of metacognitive processes and their general applicability in different fields.

It is thus crucial to explore where in the metacognitive loop—from setting goals to achieving them—the patient faces obstacles to understanding the usefulness of meta-level thinking in medical conditions. Alternatively, following Wells' argument advocating for metacognitive therapy over cognitive behavioural therapy for patients experiencing stressful events, the focus should be pinpointing gaps in the patient's cognitive control and the content of their thoughts related to their medical condition through metacognitive strategies.

In medical education, memorising, retrieving information, connecting information across disciplines, managing emotions in learning and practising bedside manners require a significant mental and emotional load. Metacognitive skills render the catalyser of all these cognitive processes. In medical studies, the research related to metacognition focusses on processing information in a problem-based learning framework [70] and not person-to-person interaction as part of transferable skills. As in any other field, becoming a medical professional requires storing and retrieving explicit and implicit knowledge. As such, one set of mental processing is given by the knowledge acquired within the medical school and another during years of medical practice through experience. Whilst this is the big picture of how a medical student follows the knowledge pathway in becoming a medical practitioner, the microscopic mental architecture involves various habits, including cognition and emotions affecting cognition. These habits are person dependent and are encountered during medical studies and in medical practice, which can be explicitly processed through meta-level cognition.

References

1. Borrell-Carrio F, Suchman A, Epstein R (2004) The biopsychosocial model 25 years later: principles, practice, and scientific inquiry. Ann Fam Med 2:576–582
2. Schramme T, Edwards S (2017) Handbook of the philosophy of medicine. Springer, Dordrecht
3. Marcum JA (2008) Humanizing modern medicine. An introductory philosophy of medicine. https://doi.org/10.1007/978-1-4020-6797-6
4. Sadegh-Zadeh K (2015) Handbook of analytic philosophy of medicine. https://doi.org/10.1007/978-94-017-9579-1
5. Marcum JA (2017) The "new" medical model, fragmented clinical care and philosophy of medicine. Can Med Assoc J 189:E897–E897
6. Marcum JA (2017) The Bloomsbury companion to contemporary philosophy of medicine. Bloomsbury Academic, London
7. Stempsey WE (2015) Handbook of the philosophy of medicine. Springer, Dordrecht, pp 1–13
8. Alfaro-LeFevre R (2020) Critical thinking, clinical reasoning, and clinical judgment, 7th edn. Elsevier Inc.
9. Cunningham TV (2013) Socializing medical practice: a normative model of medical decision-making. Doctoral dissertation, University of Pittsburgh
10. Gambrill E (2005) Critical thinking in clinical practice improving the quality of judgments and decisions. Wiley

11. Gambrill E (2019) Critical thinking and the process of evidence-based practice. Oxford University Press
12. Marcum JA (2012) An integrated model of clinical reasoning: dual-process theory of cognition and metacognition. J Eval Clin Pract 18:954–961
13. Genuis QIT (2021) A genealogy of autonomy: freedom, paternalism, and the future of the doctor–patient relationship. J Med Philos 46:330–349
14. Reach G (2014) Patient autonomy in chronic care: solving a paradox. Patient Prefer Adherence 8:15–24
15. Duncan G (2000) Mind-body dualism and the biopsychosocial model of pain: what did Descartes really say? J Med Philos 25:485–513
16. Pellegrino ED (1986) Philosophy of medicine: towards a definition. J Med Philos 11:9–16
17. Pellegrino ED (1998) What the philosophy of medicine is. Theor Med Bioeth 19:315–336
18. Engel GL (1997) From biomedical to biopsychosocial: being scientific in the human domain. Psychosomatics 38:521–528
19. Gold J (1985) Cartesian dualism and the current crisis in medicine—a plea for a philosophical approach: discussion paper. J R Soc Med 78:663–666
20. Bottaccioli F (2014) La fine della grande illusione del riduzionismo in biologia e in medicina. Epistemologia 37:5–21
21. Fuller J (2017) The new medical model: a renewed challenge for biomedicine. Can Med Assoc J 189:E640–E641
22. Gendle MH (2016) The problem of dualism in modern Western medicine. Mens Sana Monogr 14:141–151
23. Pellegrino ED, Thomasma DC (1993) The virtues in medical practice. Oxford University Press
24. Chiffi D (2021) Clinical reasoning: knowledge, uncertainty, and values in health care. Springer, Cham
25. Benedetti F (2011) The patient's brain: the neuroscience behind the doctor-patient relationship. Oxford University Press
26. Benedetti F (2002) How the doctor's words affect the patient's brain. Eval Health Prof 25:369–386
27. Benedetti F (2009) Placebo effects. Understanding the mechanisms in health and disease. Oxford University Press
28. Kaptchuk TJ, Miller FG (2015) Placebo effects in medicine. N Engl J Med 373:8–9
29. Evers AWM, Colloca L, Blease C et al (2018) Implications of placebo and nocebo effects for clinical practice: expert consensus. Psychother Psychosom 87:204–210
30. Kaptchuk TJ (2018) Open-label placebo: reflections on a research agenda. Perspect Biol Med 61:311–334
31. Flavell JH (1979) Metacognition and cognitive monitoring. A new area of cognitive-developmental inquiry. Am Psychol 34:906–911
32. Fleming SM, Frith CD (2014) The cognitive neuroscience of metacognition. https://doi.org/10.1007/978-3-642-45190-4
33. Beran MJ, Brandl JL, Perner J, Proust J (2012) Foundations of metacognition. https://doi.org/10.1093/acprof:oso/9780199646739.001.0001
34. Schneider W, Lockl K (2002) The development of metacognitive knowledge in children and adolescents. In: Perfect TJ, Schwartz BL (eds) Applied metacognition. Cambridge University Press, pp 224–258
35. Hertzog C (2002) Metacognition in older adults: implications for application. In: Perfect TJ, Schwartz BL (eds) Applied metacognition. Cambridge University Press, pp 169–196
36. Koriat A (2002) Metacognition research: an interim report. In: Perfect TJ, Schwartz BL (eds) Applied metacognition. Cambridge University Press, pp 261–286
37. Florea GP (2020) Metacognition in medicine. An interdisciplinary approach. Ann Univ Bucharest 69:81–102
38. Dinsmore DL (2017) Examining the ontological and epistemic assumptions of research on metacognition, self-regulation and self-regulated learning. Educ Psychol 37:1125–1153

39. Brown A (1987) Metacognition, motivation, and understanding. In: Weinert FE, Kluwe RH (eds) Metacognition, executive control, self-regulation, and other more mysterious mechanisms. Lawrence Erlbaum Associates Publishers, Hillsdale, pp 65–116
40. Kuhn D (2000) Metacognitive development. Curr Dir Psychol Sci 9:178–181
41. Nelson TO (1996) Consciousness and metacognition. Am Psychol 51:102–116
42. Proust J (2013) The philosophy of metacognition: mental agency and self-awareness. Oxford University Press, Oxford
43. Efklides A, Misailidi P (2010) Trends and prospects in metacognition. Research. https://doi.org/10.1007/978-1-4419-6546-2
44. Thompson VA, Prowse Turner JA, Pennycook G (2011) Intuition, reason, and metacognition. Cogn Psychol 63:107–140
45. Schwartz BL (2006) Tip-of-the-tongue states as metacognition. Metacogn Learn 1:149–158
46. Koriat A (2000) The feeling of knowing: some metatheoretical implications for consciousness and control. Conscious Cogn 9:149–171
47. Nelson TO, Narens L (1990) Metamemory: a theoretical framework and new findings. Psychol Learn Motiv 26:125–173
48. Kahneman D (2003) A perspective on judgment and choice: mapping bounded rationality. Am Psychol 58:697–720
49. Chan ZCY (2017) A qualitative study on using concept maps in problem-based learning. Nurse Educ Pract 24:70–76
50. Schneider W (2001) Metacognitive development: educational implications. International encyclopedia of the Social & Behavioral Sciences 9730–9733
51. Janet M, Shimamura AP (1994) Metacognition: knowing about knowing. MIT Press, Cambridge, MA
52. Fernandez-Duque D, Baird JA, Posner MI (2000) Executive attention and metacognitive regulation. Conscious Cogn 9:288–307
53. Koriat A, Levy-Sadot R (2000) Conscious and unconscious metacognition: a rejoinder. Conscious Cogn 9:193–202
54. Gallagher HL, Happé F, Brunswick N, Fletcher PC, Frith U, Frith CD (2000) Reading the mind in cartoons and stories: an fMRI study of "theory of mind" in verbal and nonverbal tasks. Neuropsychologia 38:11–21
55. Saxe R, Carey S, Kanwisher N (2003) People thinking about thinking people: the role of the temporo-parietal junction in "theory of mind". NeuroImage 19:1835–1842
56. Amodio DM, Frith CD (2006) Meeting of minds: the medial frontal cortex and social cognition. Nat Rev Neurosci 7:268–277
57. Meyer ML, Collier E (2020) Theory of minds: managing mental state inferences in working memory is associated with the dorsomedial subsystem of the default network and social integration. Soc Cogn Affect Neurosci 15:63–73
58. Vanstone M, Monteiro S, Colvin E, Norman G, Sherbino J, Sibbald M, Dore K, Peters A (2019) Experienced physician descriptions of intuition in clinical reasoning: a typology. Diagnosi 6:259–268
59. Lei W, Chen J, Yang C, Guo Y, Feng P, Feng T, Li H (2020) Metacognition-related regions modulate the reactivity effect of confidence ratings on perceptual decision-making. Neuropsychologia 144:107502
60. Critchley HD, Wiens S, Rotshtein P, Öhman A, Dolan RJ (2004) Neural systems supporting interoceptive awareness. Nat Neurosci 7:189–195
61. Benedetti F (2011) Seeking relief: the activation of motivational and reward circuits. In: Benedetti F (ed) The patient's brain: the neuroscience behind the doctor-patient relationship. Oxford University Press, Oxford, pp 101–122
62. Craig AD (2009) How do you feel — now? The anterior insula and human awareness. Nat Rev Neurosci 10:59–70
63. Heilbronner SR, Hayden BY (2016) Dorsal anterior cingulate cortex: a bottom-up view. Annu Rev Neurosci 39:149–170

64. Holroyd CB, Coles MGH (2002) The neural basis of human error processing: reinforcement learning, dopamine, and the error-related negativity. Psychol Rev 109:679–709
65. Frith CD (2012) The role of metacognition in human social interactions. Philos Trans R Soc B Biol Sci 367:2213–2223
66. Hart JT (1965) Memory and the feeling-of-knowing experience. J Educ Psychol 56:208–216
67. Flavell JH (1979) Metacognition and cognitive monitoring: a new area of cognitive-developmental inquiry. Am Psychol 34:906–911
68. Eichbaum QG (2014) Thinking about thinking and emotion: the metacognitive approach to the medical humanities that integrates the humanities with the basic and clinical sciences. Perm J 18:64–75
69. Sodian B, Thoermer C, Kristen S, Perst H (2012) Metacognition in infants and young children. In: Beran MJ, Brandl JL, Perner J, Proust J (eds) Foundations of metacognition. Oxford University Press, pp 119–133
70. Barrows HS (1996) Problem-based learning in medicine and beyond: a brief overview. New Dir Teach Learn 1996:3–12

Chapter 9
Metacognitive Implications on Physiological Disorders

9.1 Introduction

As conveyed in Sect. 8.3 What is Metacognition?, the working definition of metacognition refers to the explicit or implicit meta-level cognitive processes of self-monitoring, self-evaluation, self-regulation and self-control of one's cognition to achieve specific goals. Consequently, we drew upon the fact that, in medicine, metacognitive thinking encompasses these processes, but they apply differently to healthcare professionals and patients. Moreover, how these actors metacognitively process information individually affects their interactions and, thus, their relationships.

From the physician's perspective, metacognitive processing implies cognitive strategies to enhance diagnostic accuracy, optimise treatment plans and foster effective communication that may significantly affect their mental health and the patient's response to the physician's working and collaborative strategy. For the patient, metacognitive thinking pertains to the self-regulation of thoughts and behaviours in managing their health, influenced by their beliefs. In between these collective cognitive actions, there are individual processes that a patient may experience. Before delving into details, let us translate metacognition into the physiological process that generates vision as a guiding metaphor.

For an object to be seen, various actions take place: (1) the light hits the retina, (2) the specialised cells turn the light into an electrical signal, (3) the electrical signal reaches the occipital lobe where the image is then being projected, (4) this projection is transmitted at a subcortical level, the frontal lobe, through a neurological pathway (5) where, in the frontal lobe, the image is mentally processed, understood. The point here lies in the difference between seeing and understanding what one sees. As such, we are talking about the first-order process, the projection of the image on the occipital lobe through the retina and via optical nerves, and the second-order process, the mental interpretation of the seen object. It is worth noting that this

G.-P. Florea, *Metacognition and Medical Humanities in Medical Education*, New Paradigms in Healthcare, https://doi.org/10.1007/978-3-032-01070-4_9

parallel is not focussed on the eye as a sensory organ but on its neurological pathway that allows one to see an object consciously.

If we transpose this guiding metaphor to cognition and metacognition, the mental "road" on which one walks is the existence of a life-threatening problem (the occipital projection after the optical nerves send the electrical impulse from the retina) -> identifying it through cognitive processes (the subcortical level transmission within vision) -> interpreting the reaction one has within their first-order thoughts when thinking about it, thus, metacognitively processing (the frontal lobe processing towards understanding what one sees). More schematically, applied in medical practice, the process of metacognitive thinking about a physiological disorder[1] can be adapted as follows:

Physiological disorder/medical condition
(the object)

↓

Knowing about bodily changes
(cognition/first-order thoughts)

↓

Thinking about the way one thinks and feels when knowing about the changes
(metacognition/second-order thoughts)

To better understand the metacognitive implications in medical conditions, we should break down the phenomenon into first- and second-order processes. The first-order processing is the initial response to acknowledging the physiological disorder—a bodily reaction to a physical condition; the second-order processing pertains to how the patient integrates the bodily changes related to their medical condition and the impact on their well-being and quality of life—metacognitive awareness, as well as what actions they will assume in moving forward—problem-solving.

9.2 First-Order Processing

9.2.1 The Medical Diagnosis as a Defence Cascade and Adrenaline Rush Response

When facing a diagnosis, a patient may physiologically respond in different ways. One is a Fly-Fight-Freeze (F^3) reaction in quick decision-making events, and another is an F^3 response in long-term decision-making events. Both cases imply a

[1] To avoid conceptual problems regarding differences among disease, illness, or sufferance, I choose to use "medical condition" or "physiological disorder" to remain neutral to the patient's psychological and phenomenological experience.

physiological reaction to life-threatening stimuli, which causes one to take action to save or preserve one's life. These reactions are instinctive and also encountered in animal behaviour [1]. In a more detailed description, this is a defence cascade [2] that refers to the range of innate, automatically activated defence behaviours that all humans possess due to evolution. This cascade is a continuum of responses to perceived threats or danger, activated in stages, each with its characteristic neural patterns such as arousal, active defence (fight or flight), "freezing, tonic immobility, collapsed immobility, and quiescent immobility" [2, p. 264].

Arousal is the initial step in the defence cascade, where the individual becomes alert to a potential threat. Active defence is when a threat is detected; the body prepares for active defence by either fighting it or fleeing it. This well-known response is aimed at dealing with danger directly. Freezing, described as a fight-or-flight response that is momentarily paused, can be seen as an evaluation or hesitation phase, where the individual assesses the situation further before deciding on fight or flight. Tonic immobility and collapsed immobility are considered last-resort responses to inescapable threats. Tonic immobility can be likened to "playing dead," where the individual becomes physically immobile, yet fully conscious. Collapsed immobility involves a collapse of physical strength, potentially making the individual appear unconscious or dead, as an extreme form of passive defence. Quiescent immobility promotes rest and healing after the danger has passed, allowing the body and mind to recover.

The defence cascade is mediated through a common neural pathway that activates and inhibits specific components within the brain's amygdala, hypothalamus, periaqueductal grey and sympathetic and vagal nuclei. Each defence reaction has its distinct neural pattern within this pathway. Two types of physiological responses are involved: the sympathetic nervous system and the endocrine system. The changes concern cardiovascular, respiratory, muscular and metabolic changes, which affect sensory and cognitive functions and result in a behavioural response.

The sympathetic nervous system triggers one stress response by releasing two major stress hormones: epinephrine (adrenaline) and norepinephrine (noradrenaline). This neurohormone makes the heartbeat faster and pumps more blood, especially in the skeletal muscles, Whilst reducing blood supply within internal organs to redirect large volumes of blood towards the brain and muscles for fast decision making and physical strength to run or fight the danger [2]. The other stress response is neuroendocrine, with the release of cortisol, a steroid hormone. In short-term response, these biochemicals participate in a proactive response that maintains the survival instinct and life or well-being preservation by preparing the body to act and the brain to make the best decisions in that particular moment.

Moreover, cortisol is associated with memories that contain fear as an emotional state. In this way, "fear-based memories for future survival and avoidance of danger" are strengthened through cortisol discharge [3, p. 1816]. The disruption occurs when the stress is prolonged, because the response becomes maladaptive, compared with the short-term stressful events that help adapt to that life-threatening, fearful situation. According to Hannibal and Bishop, the maladaptive response includes rumination and helplessness. Besides the moments charged with fear and anxiety, these biochemicals are also released in severe pain [3, 4, p. 773].

An extreme example of a maladaptive response to a stressful event is post-traumatic stress disorder, where the levels of epinephrine, norepinephrine and cortisol are abnormal [5]. The physiological expression of the imbalance determined by a persistent or exaggerated stress response determines overall inflammation and pain [3].

Whilst animals typically resume their standard functioning after a threat has passed, humans often do not. Instead, they may become stuck in the same pattern of response associated with the original danger or trauma. Once we understand the specific neural patterns of these defence responses, effective treatment interventions for individuals suffering from trauma can be developed. These interventions aim to shift the neural patterns and, consequently, the individual's mind-body state, helping them overcome past traumas by breaking the cycle of suffering [2].

Similarly, within the medical context, we can consider that chronically ill patients face their diagnosis and medical conditions as life-threatening situations. However, the threat is not necessarily imminent but pervasive and over a prolonged period. It reflects a life-threatening condition where the required time response is longer than when the danger is imminent and has an external physical representation.

To this point, it is worth mentioning the highly cited article where Jane Turner and Brian Kelly address chronic conditions that overlooked psychological and social aspects [6]. Despite advances in healthcare that have extended life expectancy and reduced mortality from many medical conditions, the authors argue that the quality of life has not received adequate attention. This is particularly true for the emotional well-being of individuals with chronic conditions, as the associated emotional distress can profoundly impact their ability to manage their conditions and maintain overall well-being. Chronic physiological disorders can lead to significant psychological distress, including depression and anxiety, since the prevalence of affective disorders is notably higher in patients with chronic conditions compared to the general population [6, p. 124]. Diagnosing and treating depression in patients with physiological disorders is difficult due to overlapping symptoms and the complex interplay among physical disorders, medication's side effects and psychological distress. Chronic conditions often force patients to adjust their lifestyles, aspirations and employment. For some, these readjustments result in prolonged distress or psychiatric disorders. To this extent, Turner and Kelly call for a more holistic approach to medical care that integrates psychosocial support and acknowledges the importance of mental health in the management of physiological disorders.

Furthermore, Turner and Kelly highlight the importance of maintaining hope and healthy coping skills amongst patients, claiming that clinicians have the role of recognising and addressing their patients' emotional and psychological needs. They critique the notion of "positive thinking" as a simplistic approach and advocate for a more nuanced understanding of patients' emotional and psychological experiences. They bring into discussion healthcare providers' emotional toll on caring for patients with chronic conditions, with the potential for developing a burnout syndrome. In this line, they acknowledge the need for healthcare professionals to take care of their emotional and mental health to provide the best care for their patients. Increased awareness and training in the psychological aspects of physiological disorder management for healthcare providers is what Turner and Kelly consider as being a solution to the implementation of multidisciplinary care models that include psychosocial support services.

9.2.2 Patient's Cognitive Processing of Their Medical Condition

If we break down the cognitive processes involved in facing a chronic medical condition, we can distinguish between at least four stages. The first is when the patient becomes aware of having a chronic physiological disorder. The second is when possible therapeutic options are discussed with the doctor. The third stage concerns weighing the best therapeutic options and choosing the one that satisfies the patient's needs and expectations. The fourth is when compliance with the strategy is maintained.

Prima facie, because the threat lacks the life-threatening imminence character and does not have an enlivened representation, the patient can have the opportunity to think about their medical condition and how they feel about it (metacognitive). The problem that arises is that because there is not an overt education or conscious attitude in inspiring the patient to reflect on how they think and feel towards their ailment, and because the focus always goes on how to fight against it, in many cases, the patient adopts an involuntary attitude or maybe an automatic/reflex-type attitude by paralysing their mind (due to fear) with effect on thinking about their thinking, as proven in acute stress effects on metacognition [7]. Therefore, the perception of their body, how they perceive the physiological disorder, and how their life is being changed because of their medical condition are not cognitively analysed at a metalevel.

Consequently, due to animal instinct in front of a life-threatening situation, as described previously, the patients mental focus is automatically set to fighting the pathology, fleeing away from it or freezing, the patient adopting a mental representation of the ailment as one of a predator, transforming the physiological disorder into the equivalent of an enemy. Following this reasoning, the patient reduces (or is not helped otherwise) the condition of an enemy they must struggle with. Turning back to the physical reactions in life-threatening chronic medical conditions, it is clear the stress the patient is under having "to face" the enemy every day. The difference here is, as mentioned before, the time and its pervasiveness.

In the case of life-threatening external danger, the chain of physical events happens for a short time whilst mentally, the threat lingers within the victim's mind even though the danger is no longer present, evolving into a post-traumatic syndrome [8]. In the case of a chronic patient, the body lives under the same hormonal discharge, adrenaline, from the moment the patient finds out about their critical medical condition. Therefore, the relationship between the medical condition and the stress of having it is complex and bidirectional. A medical condition can trigger a cognitive stress response, which in turn can worsen the preexisting pathology. To this end, I endorse Turner and Kelly's claims over the effective management of these stress responses as being crucial for improving the quality of life and health outcomes for patients dealing with chronic medical conditions by arguing that explicit metacognitive processing is the primary cognitive tool towards an increased awareness for both parties.

9.3 The Second-Order Processing

Because of this pervasiveness and long-time confrontation with the threat, that is the chronic medical condition and the inherent implications, I argue that there is a time opportunity when explicit metacognitive processing is oriented to the best adaptive cognitive strategy towards the best health outcome and improved quality of life. Thus, metacognition can be a key factor in decision making, empowering patients to find personal resources for their best health outcome and a higher quality of life. This cognitive tool represents a solution and an add-on for the collaborative relationship with the medical professional where the patient exhibits autonomy, a cognitive empowerment that leads to action towards finding the right solution could also have an impact on health and well-being if the effect is felt on the level of stress, as metacognitive therapy (MCT) research studies prove [9]. To this extent, in the following section, I corroborate findings from three research studies that endorse this thesis' claims: *Exploring metacognitions in health anxiety and chronic pain: A cross-sectional survey* [10], *Hot metacognition: poorer metacognitive efficiency following acute but not traumatic stress* [7] and *Metacognitive Therapy: Cognition Applied To Regulating Cognition* [9].

9.3.1 Health Anxiety and Metacognition

In a cross-sectional survey, Rachor and Penney investigate the role of metacognitions about health in the relationship between health anxiety (HA) and chronic pain outcomes [10]. With a sample of 179 undergraduate students self-reporting chronic pain, the research aimed to determine how metacognitive beliefs concerning health contribute to HA and pain-related disability. The study utilised measures like the Chronic Pain Grade Scale (CPGS) for pain intensity and disability, the Short Health Anxiety Inventory (SHAI) for HA, and the Metacognitions about Health Questionnaire (MCQ-HA) to assess beliefs about biased thinking, the belief that thoughts can cause physiological disorders, and the belief that thoughts are uncontrollable.

Key findings suggest that "metacognitions about biased thinking and the uncontrollability of thoughts" predict HA in individuals with "chronic pain, while only metacognitions about biased thinking predict pain-related disability beyond pain intensity" (ibid.). The study concludes that HA and pain-related disability might not be directly associated when considering metacognitions about health, pointing towards the crucial role these beliefs play in mediating the relationship between HA and chronic pain outcomes.

This research has several implications, particularly in enhancing theoretical understanding and highlighting potential areas for therapeutic intervention—addressing metacognitive processes about health, especially beliefs about biased thinking, could be beneficial in managing co-occurring HA and chronic pain. This perspective aligns with the Self-Regulatory Executive Function model [11, p. 14–32] of emotional disorders, which posits that maladaptive metacognitions can perpetuate worry and negative health behaviours.

9.3.2 Metacognitive Efficiency in Acute and Traumatic Stress

In a two-experiment study, Smith et al. tackle the impact of acute and traumatic stress on metacognition using hierarchical Bayesian modelling, a statistical approach that allows for the estimation of individual and group-level metacognitive performance whilst accounting for uncertainty, and a transdiagnostic approach to understanding symptoms and cognitive processes beyond the confines of specific mental health diagnoses [7]. The participants involved had no history of physical or mental health issues. The authors highlight those disturbances in metacognition, which affect the ability to reflect on and evaluate one's cognitive processes, are commonly observed in various mental health disorders, suggesting a link between metacognitive function and psychological well-being. The study investigated how acute stress (short-term, intense stress) and traumatic stress (long-term stress following a traumatic event) affect metacognition. The research aimed to determine whether these forms of stress lead to changes in metacognitive efficiency.

Findings reveal that acute stress might temporarily impair metacognitive efficiency, because a correlation between heightened psychological responses to acute stress and reduced metacognitive efficiency was observed without an overall change in memory accuracy, implying that acute stress can make individuals less accurate in judging the correctness of their memories. In contrast, the other experiment focussing on individuals experiencing intrusive memories following traumatic stress found no significant alterations in metacognitive efficiency compared to controls, indicating that traumatic stress may not have a long-term impact on the ability to accurately judge memory performance, at least in the context of the specific traumatic event and its resulting psychological effects.

Therefore, Smith et al. provide evidence that adds to the complex picture of how stress affects high-order cognitive processes and mental health: acute stress can temporarily impair metacognitive efficiency, whereas traumatic stress does not have a long-term impact on metacognitive abilities related to memory performance. The findings contribute to understanding how stress impacts metacognition and highlight the importance of considering individual differences in psychological responses to stress. The implicit observations suggest that, following stress exposure, it is necessary to develop interventions aimed at improving metacognitive skills and, by extension, mental health outcomes.

At a biological level, Smith et al. outline the physiological underpinnings of the relationship between stress and metacognition, emphasising how stress responses, particularly those governed by the hypothalamic-pituitary-adrenal (HPA) axis, influence cognitive functions [7, p. 2]. Stress triggers the activation of the HPA axis, leading to the release of cortisol and catecholamines. These stress hormones play a crucial role in mobilising the body's resources to respond to stressors but also impact brain function, particularly areas involved in cognition and metacognition.

9.3.3 *Cortisol and Metacognitive Functions*

The release of cortisol has been shown to directly affect higher-order cognitive functions, including decision making and metacognition [12]. Cortisol can exert its effects on the brain by "binding to glucocorticoid receptors in the prefrontal cortex," an area critical for cognitive processes like planning, decision making and reflecting on one's own thoughts and performance (metacognition).

The binding of cortisol to its receptors in the brain leads to changes in gene transcription that can alter neuronal function [13]. This molecular mechanism suggests a pathway through which acute stress responses may temporarily impair metacognitive efficiency, impacting an individual's ability to judge their memory performance accurately. Moreover, high emotional and physiological arousal elicited by adverse or stressful events can alter cognitive processes, including memory encoding and metacognition. The physiological state induced by stress, which is mediated through changes in cortisol levels and the activation of the prefrontal cortex, may impair the ability to reflect on and monitor cognitive processes effectively. Pharmacological manipulation of cortisol, such as through hydrocortisone administration, caused impairments in perceptual metacognition independently of subjective stress [14], supporting the theory that physiological changes, rather than psychological perceptions of stress, can influence metacognitive capacity. Moreover, according to Smith et al., individual differences in sensitivity to stress, possibly due to variations in HPA axis reactivity or differences in receptor density and function, could explain why not all individuals in metacognitive efficiency following stress show the same changes.

In conclusion to this third study, the physiological relationship between stress and metacognition involves the activation of the HPA axis, changes in cortisol levels and their subsequent effects on the prefrontal cortex that can impair the ability to monitor and evaluate cognitive processes, including memory, a key component of metacognitive efficiency.

Correlating the findings from all three studies [7, 9, 10], we comprehensively view how metacognitive processes influence psychological well-being across different contexts. Metacognitive therapeutic strategies like MCT [9, 11, 15] could effectively be applied to individuals experiencing distress due to acute stress or chronic conditions of health anxiety and pain characterised by maladaptive thought patterns. Additionally, enhancing metacognitive efficiency [7] could be a key target for interventions designed to mitigate the immediate psychological impact of stress with the effect on patient outcomes.

In summary, there is a consistent theme that dysfunctional metacognitive processes—whether in health anxiety, chronic pain or reactions to stress—play a significant role in maintaining psychological distress in the process of a patient's evolution in a medical condition perceived as a stressful event or situation. The efficacy of metacognitive interventions, such as MCT, in addressing the regulatory processes of thinking offers a promising possibility for treating the acute effects of stress and the more entrenched patterns seen in health anxiety and chronic pain. The distinction between acute and traumatic stress impact on metacognition highlights the importance of context and individual differences in psychological responses that suggest a need for tailored approaches within the possible metacognitive interventions' framework.

Philosophical considerations linked to these findings can be related to one of Proust's positions, the hypothesis of the "revised memory theory."

> Constituting a person presupposes the capacity to act mentally, which in turn presupposes the ability to monitor and control one's own mental states on the basis of one's past experiences and of one's projects. For such a conscious monitoring of mental actions to occur, a specific capacity must develop over a lifetime. [16, p. 231]

According to Proust, for this to happen, one must have the capacity for self-affection and the "dynamic ability" of self-memory, which aids in reaching more desirable states.

> Thus, using a philosophical jargon, to be a self presupposes a capacity of self-affection. Self-memory is the dynamic ability of modifying one's states deliberately to reach new states that are seen as more desirable. Our claim will be that an individual's way of gaining both a self and an access to it should be constituted not by the process of recalling alone, but by being conscious of being affected, or transformed, through that very process. This new hypothesis will be called 'the revised memory theory'. [16, p. 232]

When considering Proust's "revised memory theory" [16, pp. 231–2] in the context of patients with chronic conditions, it serves as an additional aspect of Fabrizio Benedetti's findings about motivation [17, p. 103]. Benedetti identified that motivation primarily serves three roles: it guides actions towards particular goals, enhances arousal to stimulate action and arranges actions into a systematic sequence to fulfil the goal. Patients dealing with prolonged pain primarily aim to alleviate their discomfort and improve their life quality. This objective leads them to adhere to medical guidance due to a heightened state of readiness to act that may be influenced by an awareness linked to their ability to control their responses. Thus, their motivation shapes their behaviour into an organised pattern to attain their initial objective. A chronic patient aims to ease their long-lasting pain and increase their quality of life. To achieve this, they comply with the doctor's medical advice due to increased arousal, where the body is determined to act based on metacognitive determinacy. Consequently, based on this experience and their projects, their motivation directs them towards "a coherent behavioural sequence" that would allow them to reach the initial goal.

Brody et al. highlight the significant impact of the shared decision-making process (SDM) on a patient's emotions and beliefs, subsequently affecting the treatment outcome [18]. They detail how a physician presents the information and then supports the patient in selecting a treatment option that aligns with their values. This process aids the patient in making a treatment choice, which then influences their physical state through a purely materialistic mechanism and operates independently of the SDM process.

Therefore, we can conclude that a doctor's cognitive intervention can bring changes on a broader aspect, including at the patient's cognitive level, by empowering the patient in their own treatment strategy through SDM. Having said that and recalling the changes that occur when an F^3 response is suppressed, the doctor indirectly determines a metacognitive process, without naming it as such, within the patient's mind. Considering this perspective, where both patient and doctor are active in the therapeutic process, it implies the opportunity for the patients to be cognitively involved in their therapeutic process at a meta-level.

9.4 Problem Solving and Metacognition

Because second-order thoughts are considered metacognitive processes, they are linked to problem-solving situations. Davidson et al. [19] break a problem into its significant elements using metacognition as (a) the "givens," which encompass the primary conditions and variables of the problem, (b) the "goal" that outlines the ideal resolution or outcome and (c) the "obstacles," which are determined by both the intrinsic qualities of the problem itself and the problem-solver's unique challenges in bridging the gap from the primary to the wanted state.

The procedural steps in solving the problem further imply the nature of the problem, conceptualising the problem in a mental framework, planning a method of approach and reflecting on one's understanding and execution. Additionally, the variability inherent in problem-solving scenarios is influenced by the nature of the problem, the problem solver and the specific context within which the problem arises [19, pp. 207–8].

Let us consider a hypothetical case on how a patient can face life following a life-threatening experience after coming out from a coma, using metacognitive skills from the problem-solving method to see the difficulties that may arise.

9.4.1 *Identify and Define the Problem*

A first claim we can address here, even before finding the answer to this demand, is that the patient must have their cognitive abilities intact or be mentally functional with a minimum IQ before and after the coma. For such a patient, identifying the problem may mean understanding the reason for being immobilised, having been in a coma, and then perceiving or being told about the level of their physical damage. If the reason contains an emotional charge, the mental processes can be blurred until the heaviness of this load finds relief. Out of this, it is necessary to have a functional and emotional cognitive process when dealing with identifying and defining the problem. Therefore, cognitive capacity and mental health can interfere with the patient's capacity to solve the issue further.

9.4.2 *Mentally Represent the Problem*

Whilst gathering all these pieces of information, a patient may develop a different mental representation by processing cognitively in contradistinction with another patient who underwent the same type of event, having experienced similar consequences following the event itself, because "different people often represent the same problem in different ways" [19]. Davidson et al. also consider the differences between situations, as they vary with the types of the problem, the one that tries to solve it, and the circumstances when presenting the problem. How they do it and engage in it may help them, or not, in going to the next step in solving the problem, depending on the perspective they adopt.

Nevertheless, they may change how they understand the givens, the goals and the obstacles in their health problem over time due to integrating information they overlooked before [19].

9.4.3 *Plan How to Proceed*

After going through the first two stages, the patient must decide which steps and resources they can use to face their new life, a goal they set initially. Still, according to Davidson et al., the mental processes that follow are stratified into many layers and sublayers with three general characteristics: (1) it is more probable for somebody to get involved in solving a problem if it is about a novel and complex one, which in our patient's case is not only a novelty and complexity brought within their life, but also it is a matter of going further in life[2]; (2) planning is not concrete and

[2] Survival is a challenging theme if we take into consideration the significant number of studies that show the high suicidal rates [20] in chronic and severely affected patients.

complete, but more abstract: if the patient loses their reflexes and cannot move their legs and arms, and the only control that they can have is in their mind, planning will be exclusively abstract and incomplete, without being able to give it a shape on a written plan without someone's help.

9.4.4 Evaluate What You Know About Your Performance

Defined as "knowing about what you know," metacognition represents the capacity to track what one has done so far, what one is doing right now and what else is not done yet but needs to be done. It also includes the person's "control over the internal representation they have formed and still need to form for understanding and solving the problem" [19, p. 218]. In our case, they would need to evaluate their mental representation to check if it is still according to reality, namely, is it probable to achieve their goal, or do they have to change the representation or re-evaluate the goal, namely, defining clearer what facing life means to them in the current medical condition.

Corroborating what is already known about metacognition and problem-solving strategies, we can analyse clinical thinking and decision making.

Experienced healthcare providers regularly make decisions easily; in particular, they must decide over difficult situations. At the end of each decision, depending on the outcome, they ascribe a good or bad attribute to that judgment. If the result is positive, and the circumstances repeat themselves, they will also repeat that specific decision. If the marking is negative, they automatically run a self-evaluation process to determine what was wrong whilst making that decision. This inherent process is metacognitive and may be reached with or without awareness. This thought-action-effect chain changes into an automatic response or reaction that determines the easiness or difficulty in deciding over already known situations—unless other unforeseen elements change the initial setting. It then turns into rapid thinking, creating mental shortcuts, which are heuristics based, bypassing the control and regulation process and leading to automatic behaviour.

On the other hand, in unknown situations, decision making becomes an intensive mental process with a higher cognitive load. It can be considered implicit metacognition if the physician is not consciously present. If, on the contrary, it is deliberate and consciously brought, we are talking about explicit metacognition [21–23]. Whilst implicit metacognition is spontaneous and non-analytical, the explicit form is slow and deliberate. Similar to the bounded rationality theory [24, 25], metacognition, through its particular instance known as intuition, can pertain to System 1, fast thinking if implicit and System 2 (slow thinking) if it is explicit—argument presented below. Since people try to justify the reason for their decision rather than tracing the logic of their judgement [21, p. 2214], the manifestations of implicit (unconscious) and explicit (conscious) forms of metacognition prove that access to higher-order thoughts is limited and context dependent. Nevertheless, a joint action of socially shared metacognition facilitates the occurrence of explicit metacognition, as will be proven further.

This theoretical exploration of metacognition within the realm of problem solving in a medical context underscores the interconnection among cognitive processes, emotional well-being and adaptive problem-solving strategies. Thus far, I have illustrated how metacognitive skills—encompassing the identification, conceptualisation and strategic planning of problem solving—are fundamental in addressing the multifaceted challenges individuals face in a recovery stage that can be likewise applied in chronic patients. I extended the discussion to the healthcare providers in clinical decision-making processes. I highlighted the spectrum of metacognition from implicit to explicit forms and its impact on decision-making efficacy. This analysis may enrich our understanding of metacognition's critical role in individual recovery or chronic patients and clinical practice but also emphasises the necessity of fostering these skills to enhance problem-solving capabilities and healthcare outcomes.

9.4.4.1 Metacognition Versus Traditional Cognitive Behavioural Therapy

According to A drian Wells, Metacognitive Therapy (MCT) is a psychological approach that focusses on the regulation of cognition rather than the content of thoughts typical in traditional Cognitive Behavioural Therapy (CBT) [9]. MCT is designed to address a universal maladaptive thinking style, identified as a root cause of various psychological disorders, by altering patients' metacognitive beliefs—beliefs about one's thoughts and cognitive processes.

Unlike CBT, which targets the content of negative automatic thoughts and schemas, MCT emphasises modifying the cognitive processes themselves—specifically, the style and control of thinking. MCT identifies a specific thinking style, the Cognitive Attentional Syndrome (CAS), characterised by worry, rumination and threat monitoring, as central to the persistence and intensification of emotional disorders. CAS involves a cycle of worry and rumination, threat monitoring and maladaptive coping behaviours, leading to and perpetuating emotional distress. MCT aims to disrupt this cycle by changing how thoughts are experienced and regulated, focussing on metacognitive beliefs that underpin the CAS.

Metacognitive beliefs are the core targets in MCT, divided into positive beliefs about the utility of worry and rumination and negative beliefs about the uncontrollability and danger of specific thoughts. Altering these metacognitive beliefs reduces worry, rumination and threat monitoring, alleviating psychological distress.

Adrian Wells reviews evidence supporting MCT's effectiveness across various disorders, including generalised anxiety disorder (GAD), post-traumatic stress disorder (PTSD), obsessive-compulsive disorder (OCD) and major depressive disorder. It highlights significant improvements in symptoms and metacognitive appraisals, with several studies suggesting superior outcomes for MCT over traditional treatments. MCT incorporates techniques like attention training, detached mindfulness and situational attentional refocussing. These aim to develop new ways of relating to one's thoughts and enhance the flexibility of cognitive regulation, ultimately aiming to reduce the cognitive attentional syndrome and its impact on emotional distress.

Therefore, according to Wells, Metacognitive Therapy may produce a shift from the content of thoughts to the processes of thinking itself and offers a promising approach for treating a range of psychological disorders. He underscores the potential of MCT to produce lasting improvements in emotional well-being by targeting the metacognitive beliefs that underlie maladaptive thinking patterns.

References

1. Roelofs K (2017) Freeze for action: neurobiological mechanisms in animal and human freezing. Philos Trans R Soc B Biol Sci. https://doi.org/10.1098/RSTB.2016.0206
2. Kozlowska K, Walker P, McLean L, Carrive P (2015) Fear and the defense Cascade: clinical implications and management. Harv Rev Psychiatry 23:263–287
3. Hannibal KE, Bishop MD (2014) Chronic stress, cortisol dysfunction, and pain: a psychoneuroendocrine rationale for stress management in pain rehabilitation. Phys Ther 94:1816
4. Hall JE, Hall ME (2020) Guyton and Hall textbook of medical physiology, 14th edn. Elsevier Health Sciences
5. Ressler KJ, Berretta S, Bolshakov VY, Rosso IM, Meloni EG, Rauch SL, Carlezon WA (2022) Post-traumatic stress disorder: clinical and translational neuroscience from cells to circuits. Nat Rev Neurol 18:273
6. Turner J, Kelly B (2000) Emotional dimensions of chronic disease. West J Med 172:124–128
7. Smith AJ, Bisby JA, Dercon Q, Bevan A, Kigar SL, Lynall M-E, Dalgleish T, Hitchcock C, Nord CL (2024) Hot metacognition: poorer metacognitive efficiency following acute but not traumatic stress. Transl Psychiatry 14:1–12
8. Janiri D, Carfì A, Kotzalidis GD, Bernabei R, Landi F, Sani G (2021) Posttraumatic stress disorder in patients after severe COVID-19 infection. JAMA Psychiatry 78:567–569
9. Wells A (2008) Metacognitive therapy: cognition applied to regulating cognition. Behav Cogn Psychother 36:651–658
10. Rachor GS, Penney AM (2020) Exploring metacognitions in health anxiety and chronic pain: a cross-sectional survey. BMC Psychol 8:1–6
11. Wells A (2000) Emotional disorders and metacognition: innovative cognitive therapy. https://doi.org/10.1142/9789812779939_0007
12. Sladek MR, Doane LD, Breitenstein RS (2020) Daily rumination about stress, sleep, and diurnal cortisol activity. Cogn Emot 34:188–200
13. Hermans EJ, Henckens MJAG, Joëls M, Fernández G (2014) Dynamic adaptation of large-scale brain networks in response to acute stressors. Trends Neurosci 37:304–314
14. Reyes G, Vivanco-Carlevari A, Medina F, Manosalva C, de Gardelle V, Sackur J, Silva JR (2020) Hydrocortisone decreases metacognitive efficiency independent of perceived stress. Sci Rep 10:14100
15. Wells A (1995) Meta-cognition and worry: a cognitive model of generalized anxiety disorder. Behav Cogn Psychother 23:301–320
16. Proust J (2013) The philosophy of metacognition: mental agency and self-awareness. Oxford University Press, Oxford
17. Benedetti F (2011) The patient's brain: the neuroscience behind the doctor-patient relationship. Oxford University Press, Oxford
18. Brody H, Colloca L, Miller FG (2012) The placebo phenomenon: implications for the ethics of shared decision-making. J Gen Intern Med 27:739–742

19. Davidson JE, Deuser R, Sternberg RJ (1994) The role of metacognition in problem solving. In: Metcalfe J, Shimamura AP (eds) Metacognition: knowing about knowing. The MIT Press, Cambridge, MA, pp 207–226
20. Gürhan N, Beşer NG, Polat Ü, Koç M (2019) Suicide risk and depression in individuals with chronic illness. Community Ment Health J 55:840–848
21. Frith CD (2012) The role of metacognition in human social interactions. Philos Trans R Soc B Biol Sci 367:2213–2223
22. Koriat A (2002) Metacognition research: an interim report. In: Perfect TJ, Schwartz BL (eds) Applied metacognition. Cambridge University Press, Cambridge, pp 261–286
23. Koriat A, Levy-Sadot R (2000) Conscious and unconscious metacognition: a rejoinder. Conscious Cogn 9:193–202
24. Kahneman D (2015) Thinking, fast and slow. Farrar, Straus and Giroux
25. Kahneman D (2003) A perspective on judgment and choice: mapping bounded rationality. Am Psychol 58:697–720

Chapter 10
Particular Cases of Metacognitive Processing in Medicine

10.1 Intuition and Medicine

Although describing intuition is challenging due to its subtle, nonconscious and not straightforward character, attempts have been made to retrace it. Even if the researchers' purpose was to either (a) validate intuition in clinical practice [1], (b) distinguish between different types of intuitive triggers [2] or (c) determine how clinicians estimate, evaluate and use intuition [3], they made use of the interviewed physician's metacognitive skills to pursue their goals, using other related words instead of metacognitive reasoning. Thus, they pinpointed the underlying mental processes and perceptions of intuition using metacognitive processing tools. Their qualitative study was designed based on introspective interviews taken from experimented clinicians.

Intuition is the non-deliberate and non-analytical thinking felt "in the gut" as a hunch [4–7]. A person perceives these gut feelings when new variables or unforeseen elements appear. They may be experienced in already known or unprecedented situations whilst finding solutions in vital circumstances. Intuition can be seen as a higher-order instinct that enhances creative thinking and as a tool for adaptability by finding solutions to situations with little or nonexistent predictability. Through intuition, one has access to the conclusion regarding a problem and not to the complex data that may objectively justify it [8]. When intuition is taken together with explicit metacognition, the quality of that mental processing is enhanced, since the new thought is based on implicit knowledge and experience that are brought into the conscious mind and then analysed. Intuition is thus not an irrational mental process, although not voluntarily accessible, but rather a mental asset when validating the "hunch" or "gut feeling" through the metacognitive toolkit by bringing unconscious information through conscious reasoning.

I claim that two forms of intuitive thoughts can be distinguished. (a) non-deliberate thoughts, unprocessed and overtly delivered as they reach the conscious

G.-P. Florea, *Metacognition and Medical Humanities in Medical Education*, New Paradigms in Healthcare, https://doi.org/10.1007/978-3-032-01070-4_10

mind—about the System 1 cognitive process [9] and (b) covert intuitive thoughts that are first processed through mindful, deliberate thinking and metathinking processes and then overtly expressed—about the System 2 cognitive process. If the former is the "raw" form of an intuitive thought due to its subjective, biased charge, with a high rate of error, the latter is the "processed" version of the former. Those non-deliberate, unrefined intuitions fall in the processed category once they have been consciously analysed and filtered. The process that could make this processing from raw to deliberate intuition possible is metacognition. Therefore, metacognitive strategies applied to intuition may be the appropriate tools that enable one to discern between a "true" or "false" intuition, where even the conclusion of it being false is a step towards progress [10]. In this case, intuition is educated, informed, objective and, consequently, less prone to errors in the decision-making processes. At this point, we can assert that processed intuitions are informed, educated guesses, whilst unfiltered intuitive thoughts are prone to shallow thinking and implicitly to erroneous decision making. This may justify the distinct types of intuitive thinking and their relevance in medical practice [1, 2]. From this perspective, informed intuitions may be the bridge between the two cognitive processing systems. I will refer to the first category of intuitions as "raw intuitions" and to the latter category as "processed intuitions."

Using a step-by-step analytic strategy through self-reflection or metacognitive capacity, they brought the "gut feeling" to a more conscious level—see Fig. 10.1. Metacognitive processing scheme. To sum up, metacognition is a built-in human trait. If doctors disown this capacity, they will be prone to repeat the same errors in medical judgement.

10.2 Socially Shared Metacognition[1]

So far, I have presented metacognitive processes and experiences applied to the self. In this section, I discuss metacognition applied to others, also known as mentalising [11]. I claim that mentalising is a significant resource in a medical environment, working groups through collective intentionality. By mentalising, I refer to a form of the implicit metacognitive process used to monitor and predict others' mental states and, respectively, their behaviour [12].

The interaction between two or more people forms a social group. An automatic reflex activity inside the group raises a "joint action" effect where the participants coordinate their actions and bring changes to the environment [13]. If they share resources, intentions, information and knowledge whilst discussing "perceptual and decision-making processes with others" [12]. As shown above, this specific human trait facilitates the occurrence of explicit metacognition. Thus, a play between metacognition applied to the self and metacognition applied to others enables explicit

[1] Fragments published in Ref. [49].

Fig. 10.1 Metacognitive processing scheme [50]

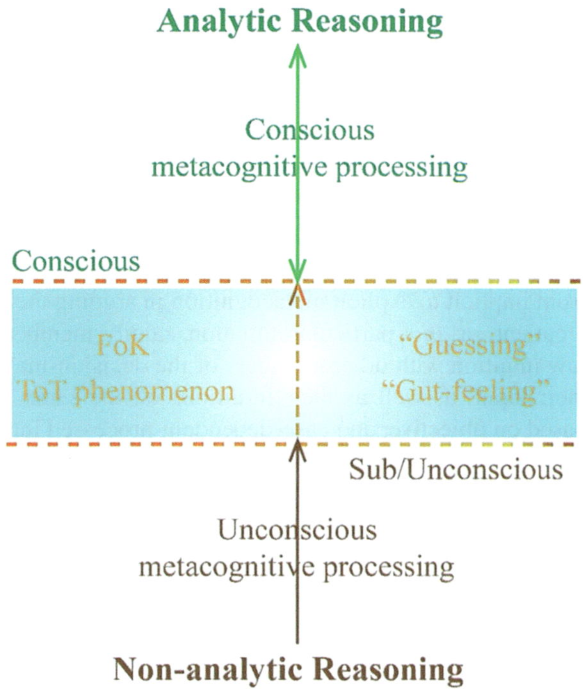

metacognition. Mentalising is inherent and essential for joint action to lead towards high performance. In other words, mentalising links minds, and this creates an effect of joint action. Joint action is thus based on action prediction, predicted effects integration, and then integrating the impact of self and others' actions.

10.2.1 In the Doctor-Patient Relationship

This intrinsic mental process makes one understand the other's beliefs and adopt a *we*-mode attitude instead of an I-mode [12]. Therefore, if metacognition is individual centred, mentalising and socially shared metacognition, the *we*-mode approach represents collective mental processing centred on the group rather than the individual. In a medical environment and any other social group, shared metacognition focussed on the *we*-mode approach has an inclusive approach to the decision-making process. The individuals who form a group decide together to achieve more than the total of each individual's results in decision making [12]. I claim that this conceptual understanding can contribute to balancing a tendency of an asymmetrical doctor-patient relationship to a symmetrical one where the I-mode of either the patient or the doctor would be replaced with a *we*-mode interaction. In other words, the idiom that the whole is greater than the sum of its parts can also be applicable in the mental activity within a medical group focussed on decision making, be it doctor-patient, doctor-family members or doctor-doctors that form the decision-making corpus.

10.2.2 In Uncertain Situations

By adopting and facilitating a *we*-mode working group approach, those involved go from implicit to explicit metacognition in arguing their opinion. Likewise, a doctor, a patient, or, in a particular situation, family members who share their subjective, raw intuition with other members of the decision-making corpus and acknowledge their input, as well as their intuitions on the same matter, an informed decision based on objective, and case-dependent processed intuitions, may be reached. This joint action between decision makers could enable creative thinking amongst all participants in the decision-making process, and those with more experience may have the chance to express their knowledge and intuition in uncertain situations. This shared intuition could be analysed and validated or invalidated by other health-care providers through complex data and the final decision to be corroborated with the patient's beliefs. Thus, the medical professional would cross from an implicit metacognitive process to an explicit one, with the support of those involved in the process. Since the basis of intuition lies in knowledge and experience, one could never be sure if the proper lesson was learned [14]. As such, the social sharing approach will be less prone to error when deciding.

In this particular situation, both parties, the one represented by the medical professional and the other by the patient or the patient family, would have their intuitive thoughts—"soft" data—checked by using analysis—"hard" data—and thus evolve from raw intuition(s) to its processed form through socially shared metacognition, implying that the final decision would be the end-result of a group intuition, let us say "shared intuition," which is greater than the physician's, based on generalisation and automatic, raw, individual intuition. Therefore, the "shared intuition" method promotes personalised decision making, resulting in a decision with a lesser probability of failure, where the quality of the physician's intuition is greater and more accurate, related to that specific person, rather than based on statistics in which that patient may not fall. I, therefore, claim that these considerations picture the ideal doctor-patient relationship. The ideal doctor-patient approach thus adopts a *we*-mode, where each of the participants involved in the clinical decision making is expressing ideas, increasing the efficiency and quality of the decision-making process, leading to a better outcome and patient satisfaction.

As stated, joint action in a social interaction determines a *we*-mode attitude that enables and enhances explicit metacognition, improving the decision-making process. In this case, certain principles must be followed for a successful medical encounter. These principles should focus on creating "social" groups where information is being shared and where the group members (the patient, family members and other medical professionals who are part of the multidisciplinary team) receive support and are empowered whilst their input is valued.

10.3 Metacognition, Intuition and Uncertainty

Thus far, I have distinguished between *raw* intuition—automatic, unconscious, unprocessed intuition, as intuition is commonly referred to—and *processed* intuition—the processed form of intuition employing metacognitive strategies in a social group that adopts a joint action approach with shared intuition implications. It is widely acknowledged that conscious and unconscious mental processes operate independently and in tandem. Neglecting one process in favour of the other diminishes cognitive capabilities. The synergy of these two systems (rational and intuitive) fosters complexity and creativity, which are inherent in thought processes. To inhibit their concurrent functioning is akin to expecting an individual blindfolded to perceive and comprehend their surroundings accurately. Intuition represents the mind's acute faculty for "sensing" potential solutions and outcomes.

Conversely, objective reasoning enhances the intuitive aspect by providing clarity and affirming or refuting perceptions. In other words, reasoning pertains to the mind's aim response, whilst intuition pertains to its subjective reaction [7]. Working together enhances reasoning whilst dividing or rejecting one another creates delusion or "paralysis by analysis" [15]. Translated into the medical context, if the physician is listening only to their intuition and is not correlating their "gut feeling" to the patient's intuition related to their own body and history, the medical professional may lose sight of the patient's needs and senses.

Moreover, raw and processed intuitions are challenged in uncertain situations. The closest relevant example from a medical perspective is the COVID-19 pandemic outbreak. It is a notable example of how fast and slow thinking processes have been explicitly manifested.

Before the outbreak of the COVID-19 pandemic, the cognitive load in medical practice was analysed by explaining clinical reasoning and decision making amongst healthcare providers or the placebo-nocebo effects. For the former instance, the research focussed on cognitive biases, heuristics and intuition, amongst others [2, 16–20]. Regarding the mental dimension within the placebo-nocebo effects, research revealed the importance of the mind-body-world interrelation [21–24] and the consequence of the patient-doctor relationship [25–28] as fundamental to the doctor-patient relationship, examined in Chaps. 6 and 7.

Due to the COVID-19 pandemic starting in 2020, the focus on the doctor-patient relationship increased [29–34], beginning with the impact that the lack of in-person human interaction had.

Intuitive medical professionals are responsible for maintaining the survival of the patient under care, with an implicit responsibility for the patient and their family members to ride the challenging uncertainties and even help for the best health outcome in turbulent times. In known and routine circumstances, decisions are reached with a light cognitive load, easy and automatic, whilst, in uncertain stances, the mental load is far above the average. It is then when the medical professional could ask for their raw intuitions to be validated, invalidated or complemented by the professional group members through available hard data or the other "social" group members' soft data, challenged over and over until the most probable decision that leads to the best outcome to be implemented further. It is then that the medical professional has fluency and rapidity in finding the best solution for the unforeseen variables that appear under uncertainty.

10.4 Discussion

As shown, metacognition represents the mental process where one mentally focusses on their thinking, known as "thinking about thinking," "cognition about cognitive phenomena" [35, p. 906], "cognition about cognition" [36], or as a "set of capacities through which one operating cognitive subsystem is evaluated or represented by another in a context-sensitive way" [37, p. 29].

On the one hand, this kind of mental activity is discussed in patients with specific neurological or psychiatric pathologies [38, 39]. On the other hand, metacognition is analysed in medical education [40–47] and in medical practice indirectly through intuitive thinking [1, 2, 48]. Therefore, one can distinguish between directly referred to as metacognitive faculty affected in psychiatric pathologies versus medical education-related metacognition and, indirectly, through intuition in medical practice as a skill derived from metacognitive thinking. Starting from this non-inclusive metacognitive applicability in medicine, I argued that the faculty of metacognitive thinking may represent a toolkit for medical practitioners and patients in mentally healthy patients or doctors. It could thus be used not only for evaluation in certain medical conditions or for medical students to store and retrieve information but also as a tool that can be used for the healthcare provider and their patients within their relationship.

The viewpoint that I defended in this chapter regards the role metacognition can play in addressing the crisis in medical care exacerbated by technological advances. These innovations have altered how physicians interact with patients and diseases, often through a lens heavily reliant on machines, sometimes overlooking the human experience within medical practice. My objective was to a priori highlight how metacognitive strategies can enhance medical practice by (1) providing doctors with new cognitive tools for a renewed perspective on patient care and (2) empowering patients to take an active role in their treatment. This dual approach is inspired by neuroscience findings and philosophical theories, by drawing from Benedetti's work on the doctor-patient relationship, by leveraging the insights of Proust et al. into the metacognitive process aiming to foster a more effective therapeutic process.

Initially, metacognitive processes were explored in developmental psychology and education. In contemporary discourse, the tendency is to bring into awareness the existence of metacognition within a mindset shaped by everyday problem-solving. To this end, within this chapter, another instance has been brought to the surface regarding long-term, life-threatening situations as a pathology can be considered from the patient's perspective. Whilst it is generally acknowledged that metacognitive abilities help one solve problems, for patients of any age with "non-educated minds" concerning survival instincts, metacognition would mean an essential key in controlling the content of their thoughts linked with their medical condition. These reactions are, of course, added to what their pathologies brought over in the first place, that is if a patient has lung cancer when receiving the diagnosis, the body will release adrenaline, also known as the adrenaline rush to stress, as in the flight-fight-freeze response; thus, the inflammation will increase as a physiological reaction to this stress hormone. Therefore, using methods that involve metacognitive processes within medical care could be beneficial during invasive (surgery) or non-invasive treatment (chemical drugs), as they could prepare cognitively the patient to manage the therapy by explicitly using their meta-level cognitive skills.

As Nelson was urging the psychologists to collaborate with philosophers to sift from fuzzy theories to those that could give a clearer understanding of how the metacognitive process manifests, I consider that the scientific forum concerned about the overall, or holistic, patient's and doctor's well-being should insert itself in this alliance to make improvements not only in what regards innovations on medical instruments/devices/artificial intelligence implementation within the medical system but also on cognitive awareness related to medical condition. Because of its multi-facet character, medicine should use theories from the philosophy of mind, neuroscience and psychology to understand the implication metacognition has on all aspects, including the patient-doctor relationship and, vice versa, the patient-medical condition relationship. Including explicit meta-level thinking in medical decisions will satisfy all levels of organisation that constitute the human being involved in this therapeutic process and have a genuinely holistic approach in medicine.

10.5 Conclusion

The end goal of this part was to offer explicit metacognitive thinking as an operational, inherent tool that a doctor can use for effective, empathetic and compassionate "collaborative conversation." Once acknowledged, this tool may contribute to developing and enhancing interchangeable skills required in any medical encounter. Although metacognition is intuitively applied to medical practice, hence implicitly, it can be consciously brought, thus explicitly, to enhance the clinical decision-making process and, consequently, to the doctor-patient interaction, with an effect on the patient's and the medical professional's mental well-being and, particularly, on the patient's outcome.

References

1. Woolley A, Kostopoulou O (2013) Clinical intuition in family medicine: more than first impressions. Ann Fam Med 11:60–66
2. Vanstone M, Monteiro S, Colvin E, Norman G, Sherbino J, Sibbald M, Dore K, Peters A (2019) Experienced physician descriptions of intuition in clinical reasoning: a typology. Diagnosi 6:259–268
3. Van den Brink N, Holbrechts B, Brand PLP, Stolper ECF, Van Royen P (2019) Role of intuitive knowledge in the diagnostic reasoning of hospital specialists: a focus group study. BMJ Open 9:1–8
4. Sinclair M (2011) Handbook of intuition research. Edward Elgar
5. Thompson VA, Prowse Turner JA, Pennycook G (2011) Intuition, reason, and metacognition. Cogn Psychol 63:107–140
6. Sadler-Smith E (2008) Inside intuition. https://doi.org/10.4324/9780203932070
7. Salk J (1984) Anatomy of reality. Merging of intuition and reason. Columbia University Press, New York
8. Sadler-Smith E, Shefy E (2004) The intuitive executive: understanding and applying 'gut feel' in decision-making. Acad Manag Perspect 18:76–91
9. Kahneman D (2003) A perspective on judgment and choice: mapping bounded rationality. Am Psychol 58:697–720
10. Wilder RL (1979) (1967) the role of intuition. Science 156:605–610
11. Frith CD, Frith U (1999) Interacting minds: a biological basis. Am Assoc Adv Sci 286:1692–1695
12. Frith CD (2012) The role of metacognition in human social interactions. Philos Trans R Soc B Biol Sci 367:2213–2223
13. Sebanz N, Bekkering H, Knoblich G (2006) Joint action: bodies and minds moving together. Trends Cogn Sci 10:70–76
14. Hogarth RM (2001) Educating intuition. University of Chicago Press, Chicago
15. Sadler-Smith E (2023) Intuition in business. Oxford University Press, Oxford
16. Alfaro-LeFevre R (2020) Critical thinking, clinical reasoning, and clinical judgment, 7th edn. Elsevier Inc.
17. Simmons B (2010) Clinical reasoning: concept analysis. J Adv Nurs 66:1151–1158
18. Victor-Chmil J (2013) Critical thinking versus clinical reasoning versus clinical judgment. Nurse Educ 38:34–36
19. Higgs J, Jones M, Loftus S, Christensen N (2008) Clinical reasoning in the health professions, 3rd edn. Elsevier
20. Hawkins D, Elder L, Paul R (2010) The thinker's guide to clinical reasoning. The Foundation for Critical Thinking
21. Ishida Y (2013) Does the placebo effect change our understanding of the causal relationship between mind and body? J Int Philos 339–351
22. Ongaro G, Ward D (2017) An enactive account of placebo effects. Biol Philos 32:507–533
23. Kradin RL (2010) Placebo response: a consideration of its role in therapeutics. Curr Psychiatry Rep 13:37–42
24. Pelaccia T, Plotnick LH, Audétat MC, Nendaz M, Lubarsky S, Torabi N, Thomas A, Young M, Dory V (2019) A scoping review of physicians' clinical reasoning in emergency departments. Ann Emerg Med 75:206–217
25. Benedetti F (2013) Placebo and the new physiology of the doctor-patient relationship. Physiol Rev 93:1207–1246
26. Benedetti F (2002) How the doctor's words affect the patient's brain. Eval Health Prof 25:369–386
27. Raz A, Harris CS (2016) Placebo talks. Modern perspectives on placebos in society. Oxford University Press
28. Benedetti F (2011) The patient's brain: the neuroscience behind the doctor-patient relationship. Oxford University Press

29. Fipps DC, Rainey E (2021) COVID-19 and the doctor-patient relationship. Focus 19:59–60. https://doi.org/10.1176/appi.focus20200033
30. Nwoga HO, Ajuba MO, Ezeoke UE (2020) Effect of COVID-19 on doctor-patient relationship. Int J Commun Med Public Health 7:4690
31. Vallelonga F, Elia F (2020) Doctor–patient relationship at the time of COVID-19: travel notes. Intensive Care Med 46:1
32. Gomes VTS, Rodrigues RO, Gomes RNS, Gomes MS, Viana LVM, Silva FS (2020) The doctor-patient relationship in the context of the COVID-19 pandemic. Rev Assoc Med Bras 66:7–9
33. Zhou Y, Chen S, Liao Y et al (2021) General perception of doctor–patient relationship from patients during the COVID-19 pandemic in China: a cross-sectional study. Front Public Health 9:646486
34. Luzet J, Beltran Anzola A, Gilibert M, Tosello B, Gire C (2021) General practitioners' experiences during the Covid-19 epidemic in the Bouches-du-Rhône department: anxiety, impact on practice and doctor-patient relationship. La Presse Médicale Open 2:100016
35. Flavell JH (1979) Metacognition and cognitive monitoring. A new area of cognitive-developmental inquiry. Am Psychol 34:906–911
36. Fleming SM, Frith CD (2014) The cognitive neuroscience of metacognition. https://doi.org/10.1007/978-3-642-45190-4
37. Beran MJ, Brandl JL, Perner J, Proust J (2012) Foundations of metacognition. https://doi.org/10.1093/acprof:oso/9780199646739.001.0001
38. Dimaggio G, Semerari A, Carcione A, Nicolo G, Procacci M (2007) Psychotherapy of personality disorders: metacognition, states of mind and interpersonal cycles. Routledge
39. Hertzog C (2002) Metacognition in older adults: implications for application. In: Perfect TJ, Schwartz BL (eds) Applied metacognition. Cambridge University Press, pp 169–196
40. Quirk M (2006) Intuition and metacognition in medical education: keys to developing expertise, Springer series on medical education. Springer. https://doi.org/10.4103/1357-6283.143784
41. Güner P, Erbay HN (2021) Metacognitive skills and problem-solving. Int J Res Educ Sci 7:715–734
42. Craig K, Hale D, Grainger C, Stewart ME (2020) Evaluating metacognitive self-reports: systematic reviews of the value of self-report in metacognitive research. Metacogn Learn. https://doi.org/10.1007/s11409-020-09222-y
43. Kuiper Anne R, Pesut JD (2016) Promoting cognitive and metacognitive reflective reasoning skills in nursing practice: Self regulated learning theory. J Adv Nurs 45:381–391
44. Chew KS, Van Merrienboer JJG, Durning SJ (2019) Perception of the usability and implementation of a metacognitive mnemonic to check cognitive errors in clinical setting. BMC Med Educ 19:1–12
45. Hamilton JH (2014) The learning of metacognitive skills through task management structures (TKS)—a new opportunity for dental student education. In: Communications in computer and information science. Springer, pp 149–154
46. Papinczak T, Young L, Groves M, Haynes M (2008) Effects of a metacognitive intervention on students' approaches to learning and self-efficacy in a first year medical course. Adv Health Sci Educ 13:213–232
47. Hayat AA, Shateri K, Amini M, Shokrpour N (2020) Relationships between academic self-efficacy, learning-related emotions, and metacognitive learning strategies with academic performance in medical students: a structural equation model. BMC Med Educ 20:1–11
48. Nalliah RP (2016) Clinical decision making—choosing between intuition, experience and scientific evidence. Nat Publ Group. https://doi.org/10.1038/sj.bdj.2016.942
49. Dumitru D, Florea GP, Minciu M (2023) Knowledge for a world of complexity: the intuitive executive and smart heuristics. In: Lebowitz J (ed) Developing the intuitive executive: using analytics and intuition for success, 1st edn. CRC Press, pp 139–158. https://doi.org/10.1201/9781032617183
50. Dumitru D, Florea GP (2023) The 'Irrational' within rational thinking: proofs from medical sciences and the arts. In: Rezaei N (ed) Brain, decision making and mental health, Integrated. Springer Nature Switzerland, pp 135–156. https://doi.org/10.1007/978-3-031-15959-6_8

Part IV
Conclusion

Chapter 11
Medical Humanities and Metacognition: Modern Medicine's Missing Links

11.1 Introduction

Medical humanities emerged in the 1970s as an interdisciplinary field integrating arts, humanities and social sciences into the study and practice of medicine to enhance the understanding of healthcare's humanistic dimensions amongst medical professionals and patients. However, the term "medical humanities" was first introduced by George Sarton in 1947 [1, p. 2]. Earlier, in 1919, Sir William Osler bridged "the old humanities and the new sciences" [2], echoing Hippocrates' view that "where there is love of man, there is also love of the art." Osler interpreted this as the union of "the love of humanity" with "the love of his craft—philanthropia and philotechnia" [2, p. 7]. The field gained significant momentum in the 1960s and 1970s, particularly in the United States, as medical schools began addressing the widening gap between patients and physicians by incorporating humanities into medical education [3–7]. A significant milestone came in 1967 when Pennsylvania State University established the first Department of Humanities within a medical school [8]. One of Europe's earliest medical humanities programmes was initiated at Hadassah Medical Center, part of the Hebrew University of Jerusalem. Initially, a pilot for the preclinical year, the programme now spans even clinical years of medical training [9].

Fragments of this chapter were published in "Filosofia Medicinei în România Post-Comunistă. De la Medicina Paternalistă la Medicina Centrată pe Pacient." In *Realitate și Aparență, Evidență și Probabilitate*, edited by Gabriela P Florea and Viorel Cernica, 55–72. Editura Universității din București.

G.-P. Florea, *Metacognition and Medical Humanities in Medical Education*, New Paradigms in Healthcare, https://doi.org/10.1007/978-3-032-01070-4_11

As for metacognition, the thinking about thinking cognitive process, it was first introduced in psychology by John H. Flavell in 1979 [10] with roots tracing back in 1965 from Joseph Hart's earlier concepts such as descriptions of "memory-monitoring processes," "tip-of-the-tongue experiences" and "feeling of knowing experiences." [11] Since then, the idea has expanded across various fields of research, including neurocognition, philosophy of mind and psychiatry, showcasing its complexity. However, its role in medicine remains unexplored aside from its intuitive aspects or indirect application in problem-based learning for acquiring biomedical knowledge during medical training.

As extensively examined in Chaps. 8, 9 and 10, metacognition is an indispensable, inherent cognitive skill that, when used explicitly, could become a powerful tool for a patient's best health outcome and for preserving the medical professionals' well-being by preventing burnout syndrome.

The connection between medical humanities and explicit, aware, metacognitive thinking represents a novel perspective on the interplay between humankind and cognition. Medical humanities programmes may be critical in developing and enhancing metacognition amongst medical students, preparing them to become effective and empathetic professionals. Before this hypothesis can be empirically tested, the following sections provide a theoretical analysis of traditional medical systems, with Romania's healthcare system as a case study, to explore the potential impact of such programmes on medical practice.

11.2 The Health System in Romania, Between 1859 and 2023

This section presents historical data only to offer the reader the context that would justify the eloquence of this chapter's purpose and does not give the work a historical character.

Following the historical thread through the notes made in the official documents between 1860 and 1910 published in *Monitorul Sanitar*,[1] we discover that doctors illustrated the state of the healthcare system at the time as "(…) their[2] Romania, a Romania full of misery and suffering, in villages or cities, of disease and death (...) a country they are trying to change"[3] [12, p. 217].

In the past, misery was defined by muddy streets, poor sanitation due to the absence of sewage systems in villages and inadequate hygiene practices across all social classes. Today, physical misery persists, although sewage systems are prevalent. Even with allocated funds for rural development, the mentality of the Romanian peasant remains a significant barrier; many resist building indoor toilets, believing

[1] The Health Monitor or The Sanitary Monitor (trans. by the author).

[2] Historian Constantin Bărbulescu refers to the medical staff of that period.

[3] "(...) România lor, o Românie plină de mizerie şi suferinţă, la sate sau oraşe, de boală şi de moarte (...) o ţară pe care încearcă să o schimbe" [12 , p. 217].

they should only be located outside the house. Additionally, some hospitals frequently fail to adhere to hygienic and sanitary standards, leading to the persistence of diseases acquired during hospitalisation.

Before the Great Union (December 1, 1918), during and after the World Wars, Romania experienced economic and political fluctuations that were also felt in public health parameters. The birth rate increased linearly despite the high number of infant deaths, and the average age increased from 41.14 years in 1931 to 48–50 in 1939 [13, p. 10].

Due to the alignment with the European Union's norms, which Romania adhered to in 2007, the European Commission periodically centralises and makes public these situations obtained from the Ministry of Health of each European country. Moreover, due to the small number of employed doctors specialised in public health, their duties are taken over by staff underqualified to the necessary competence criteria. Most of the time, problems are underreported, which is why the actual number of essential public health problems cases is unknown (i.e. the percentage of patients with nosocomial infections and those with antibiotic resistance, amongst others).

> Nosocomial pathology is an important Public Health problem in Romania due to its underreporting, low compliance of medical staff in using case definitions, acute lack of medical staff and reduction of budgets allocated to infection prevention and control in the hospital environment, exaggerated and erroneous consumption of antibiotics, generating an extremely high level of bacterial resistance, but also with the increased incidence of enterocolitis caused by *Clostridium difficile*. [14, pp. 2–3]

The report "Situation Analysis: The Annual Global Campaign <<Save Lives: Hand Hygiene>>"[4] from the National Institute of Statistics and the Ministry of Health, amongst other Romanian health bodies, highlights that nosocomial infections persist in hospitals. Moreover, Romania continues to grapple with enduring public health challenges, including high infant mortality and tuberculosis rates, despite ongoing national prevention and treatment efforts. Additionally, the country faces above-EU-average incidences of heart disease, strokes and significantly high mortality from certain treatable cancers, according to Organisation for Economic Co-operation and Development reports [15–17].

Since 2017, biennial reports from the European Commission have highlighted the challenges faced by Romanian patients, revealing the complex issues within Romania's health system [15–17]. These include a centralised social health insurance system with incomplete coverage due to the high emigration rate of Romanians who are still officially registered as residing in the country, low healthcare funding due to political and economic fluctuations, a mix of payment methods for healthcare providers, a shortage of medical staff following a significant exodus of doctors, outdated infrastructure and fragmented healthcare services. The European Commission's reports also point out concerns regarding the health system's efficiency, accessibility and resilience, noting specific problems such as the EU's highest rate of avoidable mortality amongst women, ineffective screening programmes,

[4] "Analiză de Situație. Campania Anuală Mondială <<Salvează Vieți: Igiena Mâinilor>>".

low vaccination coverage and preventable deaths that could be mitigated with robust public health measures [17].

High infant mortality remains a significant public health problem in Romania, with a rate of 7.6 deaths per 1000 live births, the highest in the EU, more than double the average of 3.6 in 2015, and more than twice the EU average [17]. Romania's life expectancy at birth ranks second lowest in the European Union [15]. At the same time, the birth mortality rate remains exceedingly high [17]. On the other hand, heart disease and stroke are the leading causes of death, whilst some cancers have sharply increased fatalities. Romania faces a significant challenge with infectious diseases, having the highest rate of tuberculosis in the European Union, including over a third of multidrug-resistant tuberculosis cases [17]. The mortality rate in Romania resulting from treatable causes is significantly higher than the European Union average, exceeding double that of the European Union [15]. Even though life expectancy has increased so far—71.2 years in 2000 and 75 years in 2015—it is lower than the European Union average of 80.6 years [17]. The same reports also evoke the exodus of doctors who chose to leave the country due to low salaries[5] and lack of social recognition, which is a critical factor in the development of the health system [15–17].

Therefore, the issues encompass material, conceptual and ethical dimensions.

11.2.1 Material Problems

The current material problems are caused by the lack of hospital facilities and the considerable number of medical staff who have left the country in recent years [18]. Shortcomings within hospitals, like the lack of efficient medical equipment and necessary medications during hospital stays, along with external hospital challenges such as quickly depleted quotas for prescription subsidies, limited access to state-supported medical investigations and the exhaustion of allocated funds, significantly hinder a doctor's ability to practice effectively. These issues not only impact the practice but also tarnish the image of Romanian doctors, undermining their professional respect and dignity.

The latest report of the European Commission (2021) shows that the real problem determining these financial imbalances in the system is how the percentages of gross domestic product (GDP) to the health system are distributed.

> Between 2015 and 2019, health spending increased on average by 10.3% per year, which is the largest increase among EU countries. In 2019, however, Romania still spent less than half the average per capita across EU countries (EUR 1310 compared to EUR 3523, adjusted for differences in purchasing power). As a share of GDP, Romania spent 5.7% on health—the second lowest among EU countries. Although the public share of health spending is high (80% in 2019) and in line with the EU average, at 18.9%, out-of-pocket (OOP)

[5] The analysis presented dates back to 2017, ahead of the significant healthcare salary increase in 2018.

> payments are above the average of 15.4% across the EU (…). Informal payments are believed to be substantial, although their full extent is unknown. [15]

Analysing further the root causes of material issues, we reach the corruption that is still present within the system and is intertwined with the political environment [19].

11.2.2 Conceptual Issues

Significant conceptual issues within the Romanian healthcare system stem from a doctor-patient relationship illustrated by a paternalistic, doctor-centred model, where communication has the most negative impact on their interaction [20–22] as well as the failure to respect patients' rights [23], the small number of doctors per capita, due to the continuous exodus of doctors trained in Romania [15, 24, 25], a fact that leads to overburdening the remaining medical staff in the country through the large number of patients attributed to a single doctor [22] or medical corruption [19, 26]. In the Romanian medical space, all these problems are intertwined due to the underfunding of the medical system, the non-implementation of health policies [27] and poverty associated with the power exercised by people who present authority in the medical, political or economic field [19], as well as the low level of education. From the scarce research on the level of dissatisfaction amongst patients treated in the Romanian medical public sector, the most significant factors are related to "medical staff's ability to communicate, medical staff's hygiene, as well as sanitary and privacy conditions within the hospital" [20, p. 7].

Other related studies are linked to the shared decision-making (SDM) process. The SDM-Q-9 is a questionnaire used widely in healthcare research and clinical practice to evaluate the implementation and effectiveness of shared decision making; in Romania, the SDM perception amongst patients reveals the valence of the doctor-patient relationship, especially in the quality of their communication. Romanian studies that have pursued these lines of inquiry show a paternalistic influence on the doctor-patient interaction [28, 29]. Patients who filled out the SDM-Q-9 survey in the hospital reported higher SDM perception scores compared to those who anonymously completed the same survey online. The authors linked it with the social desirability bias and the "avoidance of a conflict with the medical staff (…) the avoidance of negative consequences on the doctor-patient relationship and implicitly on the medical act, gaining sympathy, all due to the lack of trust in the confidentiality of the investigative act and the lack of accountability" [29, p. 7]. Therefore, inpatients were more concerned about their relationship with the doctor and implicitly the administered treatment not to be endangered to the detriment of their sincerity on the survey, because they distrust the confidentiality of the study.

The second study reveals that physicians were reluctant to disclose all information regarding treatment strategy, because the patient may disagree with their opinions as experts [28]. Some clinicians worry that if a patient disagrees with their recommendations, it may compromise their clinical experience. However, disagreements between patients and doctors may stem from a preference mismatch [28].

As for bribery, although in hospitals it is no longer a generalised practice as it used to be until recently, it is, unfortunately, still encountered in this medical system [15–17, 26], and the extent remains unknown [15–17]. Despite advancements made over the past decade, Romania still faces adverse outcomes across many healthcare sectors, mainly due to systemic issues such as corruption and nepotism at various administrative levels, insufficient funding, non-adherence to sanitation standards and inadequate public awareness efforts, despite support from European Union programmes. These challenges reflect a reluctance to embrace necessary reforms to develop a healthcare system that is economically sustainable, politically stable, and truly centred on the patient. Accountability extends beyond political or administrative leaders to include medical personnel who often remain attached to outdated practices from the communist era rather than focussing on the patient's essential needs, the healthcare profession's core.

All these problems, correlated with financial shortcomings and defective health policies, have caused a significant exodus of medical staff. The Romanian medical brain drain is "about one-third of all home-trained and native-born doctors" [18, p. 9]. Medical professionals and students who have received training in Romania often migrate to countries with more advanced medical systems due to the challenges and limitations they encounter in their home country, such as "number of beds in hospitals, the number of emigrants, unemployment rate, and income" [30, p. 1].

Political interference in the medical system is reflected in the high turnover of health ministers, which leads to little or no system improvement. Moreover, the health strategy appears promising in theory but fails to be implemented [27, p. 23].

11.3 Medical Humanities in the Medical and Educational Systems?

The primary focus of this book is on the essential role of the doctor-patient relationship and the meta-level of cognition during a person's physiological dysfunction. Specifically, this chapter provides the unique context of the conservative medical system and its particularity. Post-communist countries like Romania and Croatia, as well as low- to medium-developed countries, still follow a conservative approach despite developing a proper patient-centred medical approach [31–33]. The legacy of material shortages and ineffective policies from the communist era underpins a healthcare system where the human dimension is often neglected in practice and research. This oversight suggests that addressing interpersonal needs becomes secondary and that the critical need to prioritise humanistic concerns for patients and doctors is deficient.

As shown, the historian Constantin Bărbulescu [12] evoked the poor sanitary conditions in rural and urban settings and many Romanian healthcare facilities during the 19th and 20th centuries. A significant political phase, communism, profoundly affected Romanian society, notably shaping its medical and educational systems. It markedly influenced the transition from that era to contemporary Romanian medicine.

Today, besides its strict physical sense, "misery"[6] also refers to the figurative suffering caused by the abuse of power of certain classes, particularly affecting patients with severe medical conditions.[7] Throughout this period, the medical education curriculum did not include disciplines that would develop virtues necessary in medicine, including interpersonal skills such as communication, empathy, compassion, or management of professional stress to which doctors are exposed.

Although limited accounts regarding the experiences of Romanian patients exist, the issues within the healthcare system are well recognised, particularly by individuals who have dealt with chronic, terminal, or other forms of illness. One notable contribution to understanding these challenges is the in-depth examination of the healthcare system made by the Romanian anthropologist Vintilă Mihăilescu, titled *În căutarea corpului regăsit. O ego-analiză a spitalului*[8] [34].

The works above portray a troubling "pathology" that characterises Romania's healthcare system, illustrating its impact across various dimensions. Whilst the general public recognises some aspects of this dysfunction, the most severe demographic implications are familiar only to insiders within the healthcare system.

11.3.1 What Are the Medical Humanities?

Medical humanities are an interdisciplinary field that integrates the arts, humanities, social sciences, and natural sciences within the practice and study of medicine. Its primary aim is to foster a more comprehensive, holistic approach to healthcare that encompasses the biological aspects of illness and treatment and a person's multifaceted human experience: emotional, social, cultural, and ethical. Medical humanities offer deeper insights into the human condition, illness experience, and the societal implications of medical practices through interpersonal skills like empathy, compassion, and communication. The focus is on patient-centred care that acknowledges the patient's narrative, values and needs as integral components of effective treatment plans. Moral dilemmas and ethical issues in healthcare are central topics of debate, for they contribute to developing more conscientious and morally grounded medical professionals. It bridges gaps between disciplines, encouraging

---

[6] Sanitation in most health facilities.

[7] Rapid intervention arrangements are used for purposes other than first aid or medical care priority according to the degree of influence.

[8] "In Search of the Rediscovered Body. An Ego-Analysis of the Hospital" (trans. by the author).

collaboration amongst healthcare professionals, ethicists, historians, artists, and scholars to enrich the understanding and practice of medicine. For healthcare providers, engagement with the medical humanities can offer avenues for personal growth, self-reflection, and coping strategies to deal with their profession's stresses and emotional challenges.

Therefore, medical humanities are increasingly integrated into medical education curricula to cultivate a broader perspective amongst future healthcare professionals. The focus is on developing cultural competence, narrative competence, and the ability to engage with patients beyond their diagnoses. In this way, medical humanities integrates diverse perspectives and skills, promoting a more compassionate, ethical, and holistic approach to healthcare that values and respects the complexity of human life.

11.3.2 Humanistic Versus Paternalistic Approach

According to James Marcum, the biomedical model is framed between the metaphysical position of mechanical monism and the presupposition of reductionism and ontologically by physicalism or materialism. The humanist model is linked to a metaphysical position of dualism or holism, presupposition of emergentism and ontologically of organicism.

Within the holistic view of medicine, which Marcum associates with a humanistic approach in the doctor-patient relationship, the patient is considered a person, not an object. A *self*, or at least an organism composed of body and mind, embedded in a whole, viewed in a broader context, including socioeconomic [35]. In opposition to the holistic view, the biomedical one requires that the doctor operates with abstract, statistical concepts related to the patient's disease, not with the patient as a unique entity. Here, explanations provide information of a physical nature, with the mental aspect also being reduced to the physical level. In the humanistic approach, explanations aim to integrate psychological, social, or even spiritual determinants. Therefore, the "holistic" clinician's task is to incorporate the patient's medical condition experience into the clinical picture, encompassing the physical, emotional, and spiritual dimensions [35, p. 151], thus as a person. In contrast, the "biomedical" clinician perceives the patient only as its disease; therefore, it is an object. An in-depth analysis regarding the possible erroneous association between reductionism, paternalism, and the biomedical model, as well as between the holistic, humanistic approach and the biopsychosocial model, was made at length in Chap. 2 Gaps in Understanding the Doctor-Patient Relationship.

Whilst the physician identifies the signs of disease, specific information—known as symptoms—can only be obtained directly from the patient and not from other sources. To gather these insights, the physician must carefully consider the explicit and implicit details shared by the patient, whether through verbal communication or nonverbal and paraverbal cues. Failing to listen to the patient actively means missing out on crucial information vital for accurate diagnosis and effective treatment.

Therefore, if subjective insights blend with objective data, doctors can merge their clinical observations with their patients' personal experiences and beliefs. The results would then reflect more comprehensive and successful treatment outcomes [36, p. 97]. Robert Smith named this type of information "human data," as information communicated by the patient through words or uniquely human expressions, extending beyond laboratory data [34, p. 108].

Due to the limited attention given to these two models in Romanian medical literature, examining them in connection with research on doctor-patient interactions is crucial despite the scarcity. This exploration will enable us to theoretically identify patients' needs within a conservative medical system, particularly in a cultural context where there is recognition of an imbalance in the power dynamic between doctors and patients (see Sect. 2.1.2 Doctor-Patient Dyad Within The Decision-Making Process).

11.4 Humanistic Approach in Conservative Medical Practices

Western healthcare systems have shifted from a doctor-centred approach to patient autonomy through empowerment. Whilst achieving a similar change in conservative countries like Romania may pose challenges due to the entrenched practice of doctor-centred medicine, the following sections theoretically explore approaches in this direction.

11.4.1 Marcum's Argument

To provide proper medical care, a physician must understand a patient's ethical and aesthetic principles and the medical condition's scientific attributes [35]. One can fully understand the clinical picture by considering the relationship between patient and doctor in a unified and humanistic context. Therefore, the clinician must be open to these two complex perspectives to have a holistic picture of the patient's condition. This attitude aims to provide a complete medical record of the patient's treatment and/or cure.

> Even though medicine is a social enterprise and is influenced by larger social (political, economic, cultural, and religious) values and goals, its central relationship is narrowly defined in terms of the patient-physician relationship (...) It is this relationship that is one of the most important elements in defining the very nature of medicine itself, since medicine is therapeutic at its core. [35, pp. 108–9]

When the doctor focusses on the patient's human aspects through active listening, they gain critical insights not only into the patient's personal experiences but also into the progression of the disease. For a doctor adhering strictly to mechanistic biomedical precepts, such nuanced information remains inaccessible if the data from clinical investigations do not change. Thus, Marcum highlights that the absence of a more holistic approach amongst doctors strictly adhering to the biomedical view favoured a decline in healthcare quality. To address this ongoing global crisis, Marcum underscores the importance of adopting the holistic view, hence the humanistic approach. This approach aims to enrich patients' lives, particularly vital for those with chronic or terminal conditions, by emphasising care that goes beyond mere physical healing (ibid.). Patients expect a doctor to treat the diseased body and the *person* suffering from the disease. At the same time, Marcum highlights that humanist/humane medicine does not give up scientifically validated proven treatments but wants to reach a cure through ethos [35, p. 276].

> Within an ethos of care, a physician is no longer the locus of supreme authority and power in curing patients but a first-among-equals co-participant with them. The physician then recognizes that the patient's body/mind often cures itself and that the role of both the physician and the patient is to assist in that process and not to hinder it. The patient-physician relationship is one of mutual respect, for the role and contribution of each other in the curing process. [35, pp. 108–9]

11.4.2 Pellegrino's Argument

Edmund Pellegrino seeks to establish the foundations of physicians' obligations by examining the nature of medicine itself [37]. He aims to provide a new side of what the doctor-patient relationship should represent, starting from what Scribonius Largus was trying to establish in the first century AD as a physician to Emperor Claudius. Therefore, Pellegrino brings to attention the two principles underpinning the practice of medicine at that time: *humanitas* and *misericordia. Humanitas* as kindness directed towards humanity, different from *philanthropy*—benevolence for the benefit of poor people—and *misericordia* as compassion for the sick.

Moreover, he proposes to elaborate a concept in medical practice based on a philosophical foundation to outline medical professionals' obligations through an analysis of the nature of the patient-doctor relationship. In developing this idea, he invokes three phenomena that need to be considered: (1) suffering, (2) the act of profession and (3) the medical act.

As for *suffering*, according to Pellegrino, it occurs when the individual realises that he needs help, following symptoms that they consider threatening. The most suggestive example is the case of a person who experiences chest pain and, because they assume a life-threatening heart condition, decides to seek medical attention; thus, suffering occurs only when the person decides to be consulted by a specialist. The moment of awareness or recognition of deviations from the state of health and, at the same time, the person's decision to be consulted by a specialist constitutes the onset of suffering. Because of this suffering, Pellegrino believes a rupture occurs between the patient's body and *self.* Before this physiological imbalance that brings the individual into a state of suffering, the body was an instrument they could easily use; now, the body turns into a tyrant with demands that must be listened to and taken where necessary to receive attention and help.

Apart from this rupture, the affected person loses part of their freedom and wants to know the answers to three fundamental questions about the state in which they find themselves: "*What's wrong? What can be done?* and *What ought to be done?*" [37, p. 67].

Therefore, the previously independent person becomes vulnerable, a patient and forced to leave themselves in the hands of the one who can offer help. The rhetorical question that involuntarily arises in a patient's mind and that Pellegrino presents, *"Is this the beginning of the end of my existence?"* reflects the state of panic or fear of death that the sufferer experiences due to the fragility generated by the affectation from which they suffer. In this state of vulnerability, the *act of the profession* comes into question, the second element enunciated by Pellegrino, as part of the patient-doctor relationship. Pellegrino describes the unequal power dynamic between doctor and patient, as the patient seeks help from the doctor who provides it based on their knowledge and experience.

Finally, *the medical act* is the third element of the patient-doctor relationship, as outlined by Pellegrino. Through it, the doctor gets involved in those actions that lead to a correct decision to heal the patient: to reunite the patient, restore harmony and, if possible, to be able to do it even better than it was before the suffering set in. Pellegrino distinguishes between a healing decision and a good one. The healing decision implies scientific knowledge, making it "a medical competent decision," whilst a good decision implies considering various factors, including age, current situation, aspirations, expectations and values. All these constitute the integral to their identity, and it is therefore critical to understand what is in their own interest [37, p. 67].

11.4.3 Pellegrino's Counterargument to Paternalism

In the same work, Pellegrino dismantles the image perpetuated over time and universally accepted without being questioned since Hippocrates' times [37]. This image gives the doctor the attribute of an authoritative person who decides for the patient what is best for him or her. Even though this attitude was useful to humanity in those times, it can no longer be applied in our era in any developed country, including Romania.

> That image is of the physician as a benign, benevolent, all-knowing authoritarian figure who decides what is best for his patients. That conception served humanity well in a time that was simpler and when medical decisions did not involve, as they do increasingly today, a host of new questions of values and morality it more easily fulfilled expectations in a society in which there were very few educated people who would say, "Just a moment—I would like to understand what is happening! I want to have a say in what you are going to do. [37, p. 66]

Through this perspective, Pellegrino challenges the principles of the Hippocratic Corpus because of the authoritarian, paternalistic and omniscient image created around doctors. This image can no longer be maintained today in a democratic, pluralistic society where access to information is limitless.

Although more than two millennia have passed since the Hippocratic Corpus postulated the role and attributes of the doctor, in conservative countries like Romania, this obsolete understanding of the doctor-patient relationship is still present without a clear tendency to adapt to the patient's evolution concerning their knowledge and access to it.

11.4.4 "Adam U'Refuah" Argument

Through the *Adam U'Refuah*[9] *Medical Humanities* programme, the Faculty of Medicine of the Hebrew University of Jerusalem has contributed to developing and enhancing future physicians' ability to use scientific knowledge empathetically and humanely. The overall goal was to remind students that medicine is not within the boundaries that define disease from a biological point of view but also involves a philosophical perspective common to those who remain committed to the art of being a doctor [9, p. 307].

The concept of medical humanities was used starting from Martyn Evans' [3] definition as "an integrated, interdisciplinary, philosophical approach to recording and interpreting human experiences of illness, disability, and medical intervention, encompassing fields within the arts, humanities, and social sciences" [9, p. 309].

The programme was applied to the first 3 years of study, part of the preclinical segment of medical studies. Humanities subjects taught in this programme were related to:

> [M]edical issues in culture, such as the philosophical basis of decision making, narrative medicine, shifting attitudes to death in Western culture, anthropological and historical aspects of medical reasoning; others are of a more general nature, relating to medicine through their subtle emotional and associative effects, such as medicine and the visual arts, medicine and music, and literary portrayals of suffering and sickness. [9, p. 311]

Shaham et al. regard the "doctor-patient communication, cultural competency and professionalism to be taught in a pre-planned, comprehensive way (…) to small groups of students by an interdisciplinary staff, with immediate application during an early clinical exposure" [9, p. 311]. Therefore, the main goal of the programme was to develop communication skills. For this, students were guided and monitored in dialogue with standardised patients,[10] observed by a physician and colleagues

[9] Translated from Hebrew to English as "the human being and medicine" [9 , p. 309].

[10] Standardised patients are individuals trained to simulate patients or characters in medical education [38].

who offered their feedback at the end. This teaching method encouraged student participation and built strong relationships with their teachers.

Despite their busy clinical and research programmes, the academics who participated in supporting the educational plan were very many. Moreover, one of the conclusions they reached was that the impact their involvement in this medical humanities programme had on them made them realise that it was necessary for future doctors as well as for faculty members who taught the proposed courses.

After the success of this three-year pilot programme for the 2007–2010 preclinical years, the Jerusalem Faculty of Medicine decided to continue it. Since 2019, the Medical *Humanities curriculum* covers preclinical and clinical years. Thus, 12 years after the introduction of humanities in the faculty of medicine, the programme was extended to 5 years. In this way, medical students are trained to become not only good professionals in understanding physiological and pathophysiological mechanisms but also humans in the art they profess, good listeners and able to communicate at the level of each type of patient.

11.5 Discussion

It is an understatement to say that medical practice is not a static process between a patient and a physician and evolves according to society's changes and its direction of development. Medicine without a patient does not exist. Continuously proving that the focus should be on the patient becomes obsolete, pointless and even superfluous. Instead, attention should be placed on preparing future doctors to establish healthy relationships with their patients and colleagues for the patients' best health outcomes. In this vein, the question would be: "Is it necessary to have models for approaching patients, or would mentality change help develop further a medicine centred on human-to-human interaction?" The change in mentality would consist of the assumption of responding to the current needs of the modern patient. If these needs are not considered, they may generate and further perpetuate the "crisis of the quality of medical care," overburdening the medical personnel.

Implementing a programme focussed on studying medical humanities and extending it from 3 to 5 years at the Faculty of Medicine of the Hebrew University of Jerusalem proves that there is a concrete plan for an ongoing patient-centred medical practice. This approach determines a true humanistic mindset amongst future medical doctors who study at this university, because education is the foundation of mentality changes. The need for a common space between medicine as a science and art is felt especially by patients and medical professionals whose level of empathy naturally exceeds the norm. Once trained to observe the patient's needs, not only their disease, through active listening and learning, any doctor can increase their professional success rate by gathering more information from the dialogue with the patient. All gathered information constitutes the elements that compose the integral identity, critical to understanding what is in the patient's best interest.

The problems caused by the lack of high-performance facilities and medical personnel shortages within Romanian medical centres are not negligible. Acknowledging the flaws expressed in the doctor-patient relationship demands the same priority.

Research concerning patients' and students' needs in the conservative Romanian medical and educational systems must be pursued to understand better what aspects should be worked on. Accordingly, a plan tailored to these needs should be developed for implementation within the Romanian medical faculties. In this way, the humanities will have a targeted application to the specific problems of the local academic and hospital environment. A possible perspective could encompass patients' respect for medical personnel due to a relationship developed naturally on mutual trust. Consequently, paternalism could be gradually replaced with relationship-centredness, generation after generation.

Hence, the long-term outcomes aim to transform both the academic and professional environments by fostering a medical community that prioritises human values alongside scientific rigor. This shift could potentially discourage the migration of Romanian medical staff and patients to other medical systems. Patients would develop greater trust in doctors who could excel in managing their relationships. This emphasis on professional skills, respect and dignity within Romania would serve as added value in patient care.

Therefore, cultivating the qualitative skills essential for a modernised medical system centred on the patient-doctor relationship involves transforming the outdated paternalistic approach that could entail shifting from a rigid mentality confined within specific models or patterns to adaptive approaches tailored to the patient's needs and context. Future doctors could thus apply scientific and technical knowledge empathetically, recognising that medicine extends beyond biology and technology, encompassing human values. Addressing the patient's emotional aspects within their medical condition requires a shared philosophical perspective amongst doctors dedicated to the art of medicine: prioritising patient relationships and treatment rooted in human values, not solely biological ones.

If respect and the quality of human interrelationships in the medical community register a qualitative leap, then society's voice, on an extended level, will be able to constrain the political class in regulating and implementing the necessary changes for a healthy healthcare system regardless of its technical deficiencies. The need for doctors trained in the national educational system to leave their country of origin could significantly decrease, and patients' access to the health system will be eased by a greater number of doctors per capita.

A shift in mentality would lead to a shift in attitude and, therefore, a balanced approach towards patients. The vicious circle rooted in the communist period could be broken, and the opportunity for the system to thrive would rise. Therefore, restating humanity through a sane doctor-patient relationship in a conservative medical system would trigger physicians to want to make a change for the benefit of this system and not choose the migration route. Implicitly, a significant impact would be on the general population's benefit.

The system is made up of people. People make the policies and determine their implementation. When they choose to leave, the community power they belong to diminishes, as does the system they form. Therefore, Romanian medical professionals would find it difficult to abandon their professional *home* once they feel that the beliefs of the medical system they stepped into once they chose the path of practicing medicine share the same values as their *own* belief system, that of being able and let to provide their help for the benefit of suffering people. For all these changes to take place, one needs to be metacognitively aware of their metacognitive feelings when practicing in the current Romanian medical system and observe how their mind's extension into this clinical setting actually influences it, as well as the interaction with their patients.

11.6 Conclusion

This final chapter aimed to build a persuasive case for embedding medical humanities within the medical curriculum, especially in medical-conservative countries like Romania. In a sense, an educational reformation, given by the integration of humanistic disciplines in medical education, could be a catalyst for a mentality shift from a predominantly paternalistic model of care to one that is patient-centred through a healthy doctor-patient relationship. The chapter underscored the multifaceted benefits of this approach drawing on historical analyses, philosophical arguments and case studies (e.g. the successful integration of humanities in medical education at the Hebrew University of Jerusalem).

Through a determined effort to prioritise human values in medical education and practice, the arguments presented underlined a future where the Romanian medical community is empowered to resist the lure of migration fostering a more trusting and respectful healthcare environment for both practitioners and patients.

In addition, the discussion section highlighted the metacognitive tool accessible to every medical professional, a tool enabling them to monitor their cognitive load whilst addressing the complexities inherent in this imperfect system. This meta-level approach, which necessitates individual engagement, holds the potential to disrupt the cycle perpetuated by a flawed system in which they are integral components. By addressing the problem at its root—the medical education system—establishing medical humanities programmes to develop and enhance metacognitive thinking in medicine fosters the re-integration of humanity into modern medical practice. These efforts can mitigate the "quality-of-care crisis," sustain humanism in healthcare and balance the demands of a technology-driven era whilst improving the well-being of both patients and medical professionals.

References

1. McFarland J, Markovina I, Gibbs T (2018) Opening editorial—the importance of the humanities in medical education. MedEdPublish 7:140

2. Osler W (1919) The old humanities and the new science. BMJ 2:1–7
3. Evans M (2002) Reflections on the humanities in medical education. Med Educ 36:508–513
4. Macnaughton J (2000) The humanities in medical education: context, outcomes and structures. Med Humanit 26:23–30
5. Kollmer Horton ME (2019) The orphan child: humanities in modern medical education. Philos Ethics Humanit Med 14:1–6
6. Carson RA (2006) Public expectations and physicians' responsibilities: voices of medical humanities. Ann Intern Med. https://doi.org/10.7326/0003-4819-144-7-200604040-00026
7. Bates V, Bleakley A, Goodman S (2014) Medicine, health and the arts. Approaches to the medical humanities. Routledge
8. Allen P (2023) What are the medical humanities? Perlego. https://www.perlego.com/knowledge/study-guides/what-are-the-medical-humanities/?utm_source=chatgpt.com. Accessed 9 Jan 2024
9. Shaham D, Kandel L, Gural A (2011) Establishing a medical humanities program in Israel: challenges and solutions. Eur Leg 16:307–315
10. Flavell JH (1979) Metacognition and cognitive monitoring. A new area of cognitive-developmental inquiry. Am Psychol 34:906–911
11. Hart JT (1965) Memory and the feeling-of-knowing experience. J Educ Psychol 56:208–216
12. Bărbulescu C (2015) România medicilor: medici, ţărani şi igienă rurală în România de la 1860 la 1910. Humanitas
13. Setlacec D (1998) Medicina românească-medicină europeană: 1918–1940. Humanitas
14. (2015) Analiză de situaţie. Campania Anuală Mondială „Salvează vieţi: Igiena Mâinilor"
15. OECD EO on HS and P (2021) Romania: country health profile 2021. OECD Publishing, Brussels
16. OECD EO on HS and P (2019) Romania: country health profile 2019. OECD Publishing, Brussels
17. OECD EO on HS and P (2017) Romania: Country Health Profile 2017. https://doi.org/10.1787/9789264283534-en
18. OECD.ContributionofmigrantdoctorsandnursestotacklingCOVID-19crisisinOECDcountries. 2020.; https://www.oecd.org/coronavirus/policy-responses/contribution-of-migrant-doctors-and-nurses-to-tackling-covid-19-crisis-in-oecd-countries-2f7bace2/#section-d1e1830.
19. Ungureanu MI, Gheorghe A, Voinea ŞA (2017) Patients are denied care because of corruption in Romania. Lancet 390:2139
20. Popa D, Druguş D, Leaşu F, Azoicăi D, Repanovici A, Rogozea LM (2017) Patients' perceptions of healthcare professionalism—a Romanian experience. BMC Health Serv Res 17:463
21. Hanganu B, Manoilescu IS, Paparau C, Gheuca-Solovastru L, Buhas CL, Szalontay AS, Ioan BG (2022) Why are patients unhappy with their healthcare? A Romanian physicians' perspective. Int J Environ Res Public Health. https://doi.org/10.3390/IJERPH19159460
22. Petre I, Barna F, Gurgus D, Tomescu LC, Apostol A, Petre I, Furau C, Năchescu ML, Bordianu A (2023) Analysis of the healthcare system in Romania: a brief review. Healthcare. https://doi.org/10.3390/HEALTHCARE11142069
23. Nanu CA, Plaiasu MC, Edu A (2023) Geographic and specialty-specific disparities in physicians' legal compliance: a national-scale assessment of Romanian medical practice. Healthcare (Switzerland). https://doi.org/10.3390/HEALTHCARE11040499/S1
24. Spiru L, Traşcu RI, Turcu I, Mărzan M (2011) Perpetual transitions in Romanian healthcare. EPMA J 2:341
25. Suciu ŞM, Popescu CA, Ciumageanu MD, Buzoianu AD (2017) Physician migration at its roots: a study on the emigration preferences and plans among medical students in Romania. Hum Resour Health 15:1–9
26. Slot B, Weistra K, Oortwijn W, Van Wanrooij N, Raets T (2017) Updated study on corruption in the healthcare sector: final report. https://doi.org/10.2837/68580
27. Meijer EJC (2019) The Romanian health care sector, commercial opportunities and possibilities for cooperation. Netherlands Enterprise Agency, Hague

28. Paduca A, Arnaut O, Beschieru E, Lundmark PO, Bruenech JR (2021) Shared decision making and patients satisfaction with strabismus care—a pilot study. BMC Med Inform Decis Mak 21:1–10
29. Baicus C, Balanescu P, Zeh S et al (2019) Characteristics of shared decision making in Romania from the patient perspective: a cross-sectional multicentric study. J Eval Clin Pract 25:1152–1159
30. Apostu SA, Vasile V, Marin E, Bunduchi E (2022) Factors influencing physicians migration—a case study from Romania. Mathematics 10:505
31. Murgic L, Hébert PC, Sovic S, Pavlekovic G (2015) Paternalism and autonomy: views of patients and providers in a transitional (post-communist) country. BMC Med Ethics. https://doi.org/10.1186/S12910-015-0059-Z
32. Málaga G, Romero ZO, Málaga AS, Cuba-Fuentes S (2017) Shared decision making and the promise of a respectful and equitable healthcare system in Peru. Z Evid Fortbild Qual Gesundhwes 123–124:81–84
33. Florea GP (2019) Philosophy of medicine in post-communist Romania. From a paternalistic model toward a patient-centered medicine. In: Florea GP, Cernica V (eds) Reality and appearance, evidence and probability. University of Bucharest Publishing House, Bucharest, pp 55–72
34. Mihăilescu V (2019) În căutarea corpului regăsit. Polirom
35. Marcum JA (2008) Humanizing modern medicine. An introductory philosophy of medicine. https://doi.org/10.1007/978-1-4020-6797-6
36. Davis-Floyd R, St. John G (1998) From doctor to healer: the transformative journey. Rutgers University Press, New Brunswick
37. Pellegrino ED (2006) Toward a reconstruction of medical morality. Am J Bioeth 6:65–71
38. Battles JB, Wilkinson SL, Lee SJ (2004) Using standardised patients in an objective structured clinical examination as a patient safety tool. Qual Saf Health Care 13:i46–i50

Glossary

Bedside (medicine) The clinical practice environment where direct doctor-patient interaction occurs, involving diagnosis, treatment, communication and the human aspects of care delivery.

Bench (medicine) The domain of biomedical research conducted in laboratories, focussing on molecular, cellular and genetic mechanisms of disease, often forming the basis of translational research.

Biomedical (model) A framework that explains health and illness primarily through biological factors, focussing on physical processes such as pathology, biochemistry and physiology, often excluding psychological or social influences.

Biopsychosocial (model) An integrative model of medicine that considers biological, psychological and social factors as jointly influencing health, illness and treatment outcomes.

Doctor-patient binom/dyad The relational and communicative dynamic between a doctor and a patient, often framed as a dual structure influencing diagnosis, trust and therapeutic decision making.

Extended mind A philosophical concept proposing that cognitive processes can extend beyond the individual's brain and body, incorporating tools, environment and social interactions as part of thinking.

Explicit metacognitive awareness The conscious and deliberate ability to reflect on, monitor and regulate one's own thought processes. It involves intentional recognition of cognitive strategies, evaluation of understanding and active adjustment of thinking, often verbalised or reported. Especially relevant in clinical reasoning and reflective practice.

Humanistic (medicine) A model of medical practice that emphasises patient-centred and relationship-centred care, empathy, meaning and respect for the subjective experience of illness, in contrast to reductionist approaches.

Humanity The quality of compassion, ethical awareness and recognition of the patient as a person, integral to humanistic and relational models of care.

G.-P. Florea, *Metacognition and Medical Humanities in Medical Education*, New Paradigms in Healthcare, https://doi.org/10.1007/978-3-032-01070-4

Implicit metacognitive awareness The non-conscious or automatic regulation of thinking processes that occurs without deliberate reflection. It includes intuitive adjustments in problem solving or decision making, often based on experience or familiarity, without the individual being fully aware of the underlying cognitive strategies.

Medical humanities An overarching umbrella that includes disciplines such as philosophy, literature, ethics and history to enrich medical practice and education by deepening understanding of the human aspects of healthcare.

Metacognition The cognitive capacity to reflect on and regulate one's own thought processes, commonly described as "thinking about thinking." It involves self-monitoring, self-evaluation and self-regulation of cognition, and is especially relevant in clinical reasoning, decision making and reflective practice in healthcare.

Paradigm shift A fundamental change in the underlying concepts, practices or values of a scientific discipline, often triggered by new discoveries or philosophical critiques.

Paternalistic (medicine) A traditional model of medical care where the doctor makes decisions on behalf of the patient, assuming a guiding or controlling role, often without shared decision making.

Placebo A substance or intervention, including the medical ritual, with no intrinsic therapeutic effect, used in clinical practice or research to assess the efficacy of active treatments.

Placebo effect A psychological and physiological response to an inactive substance or intervention, based on the patient's expectations of benefit.

Placebo response The overall beneficial outcome following the administration of a placebo, which may include spontaneous improvement, regression to the mean or psychological effects.

Problem solving A cognitive process involving analysis, decision making and the implementation of strategies to resolve certain challenges.

Semantic relationism A conceptual framework adapted from Kit Fine's theory, used to analyse the doctor-patient relationship by viewing both doctor and patient as variables whose meanings and roles depend on their intrinsic (internal) features and extrinsic (relational) dynamics within a medical encounter.

Index

G.-P. Florea, *Metacognition and Medical Humanities in Medical Education*, New Paradigms in Healthcare, https://doi.org/10.1007/978-3-032-01070-4

GPSR Compliance

The European Union's (EU) General Product Safety Regulation (GPSR) is a set of rules that requires consumer products to be safe and our obligations to ensure this.

If you have any concerns about our products, you can contact us on ProductSafety@springernature.com

In case Publisher is established outside the EU, the EU authorized representative is:

Springer Nature Customer Service Center GmbH
Europaplatz 3
69115 Heidelberg, Germany

Batch number: 08826958

Printed by Printforce, the Netherlands